Color!

Mandala Mama

Deb Gilbert

Heller Brothers Publishing

Title: Color! Mandala Mama
Author: Deb Gilbert
Published by: Heller Brothers Publishing

Copyright © 2016 by Deb Gilbert
Photo Credits: karakotsya@depositphotos.com
First Edition, 2016
Published in USA

ISBN 978-1-944678-08-1

ISBN 9781944678081

90000 >

9 781944 678081

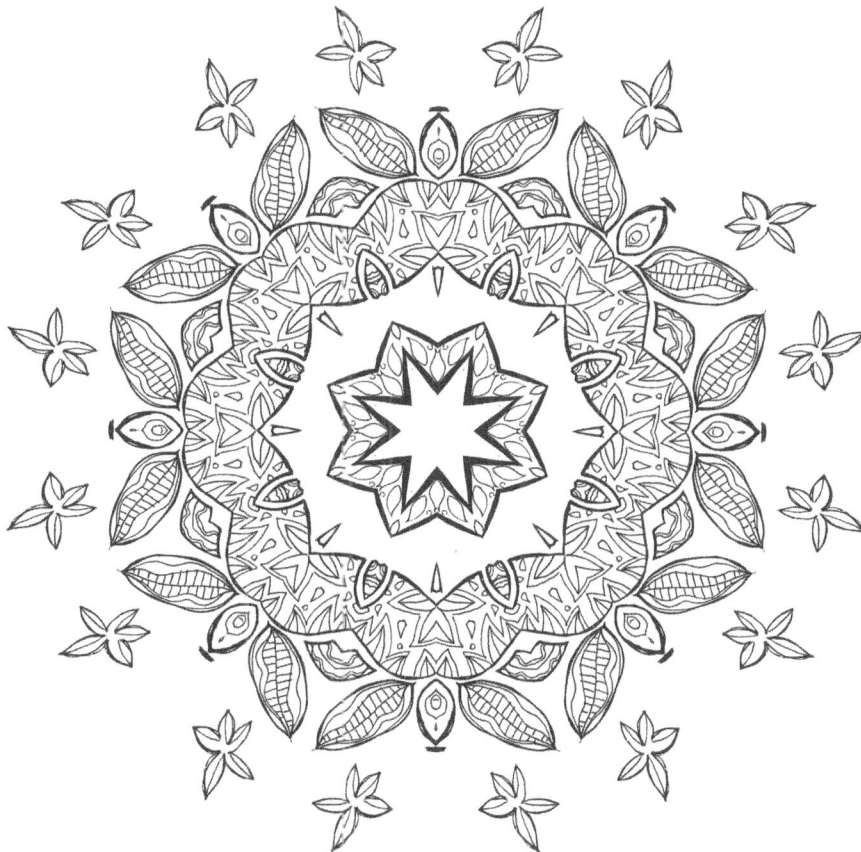

This Coloring Book Belongs To:

_____

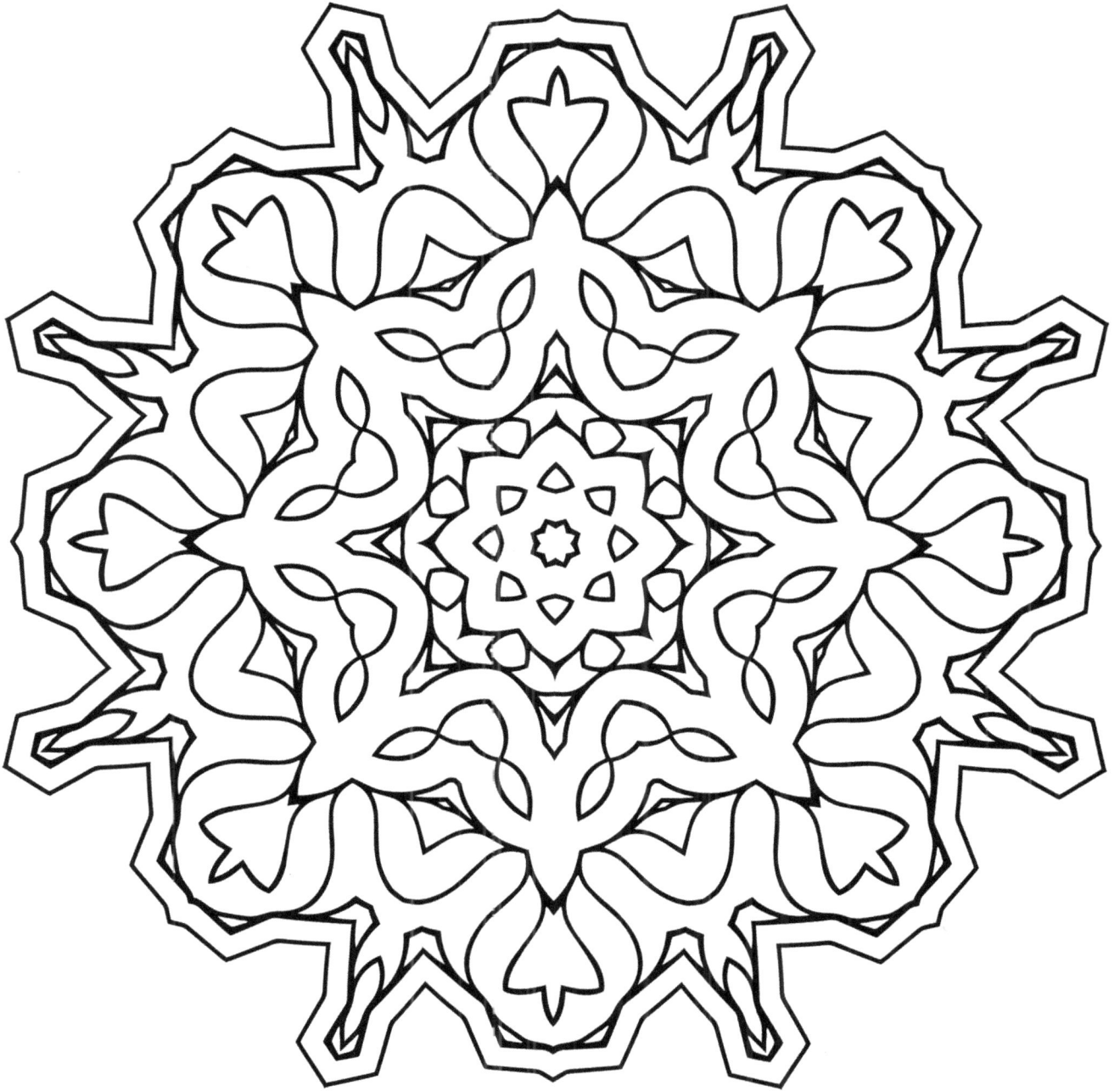

Date Completed: _____

Media Used:_____

_____

_____

Notes: _____

_____

_____

_____

_____

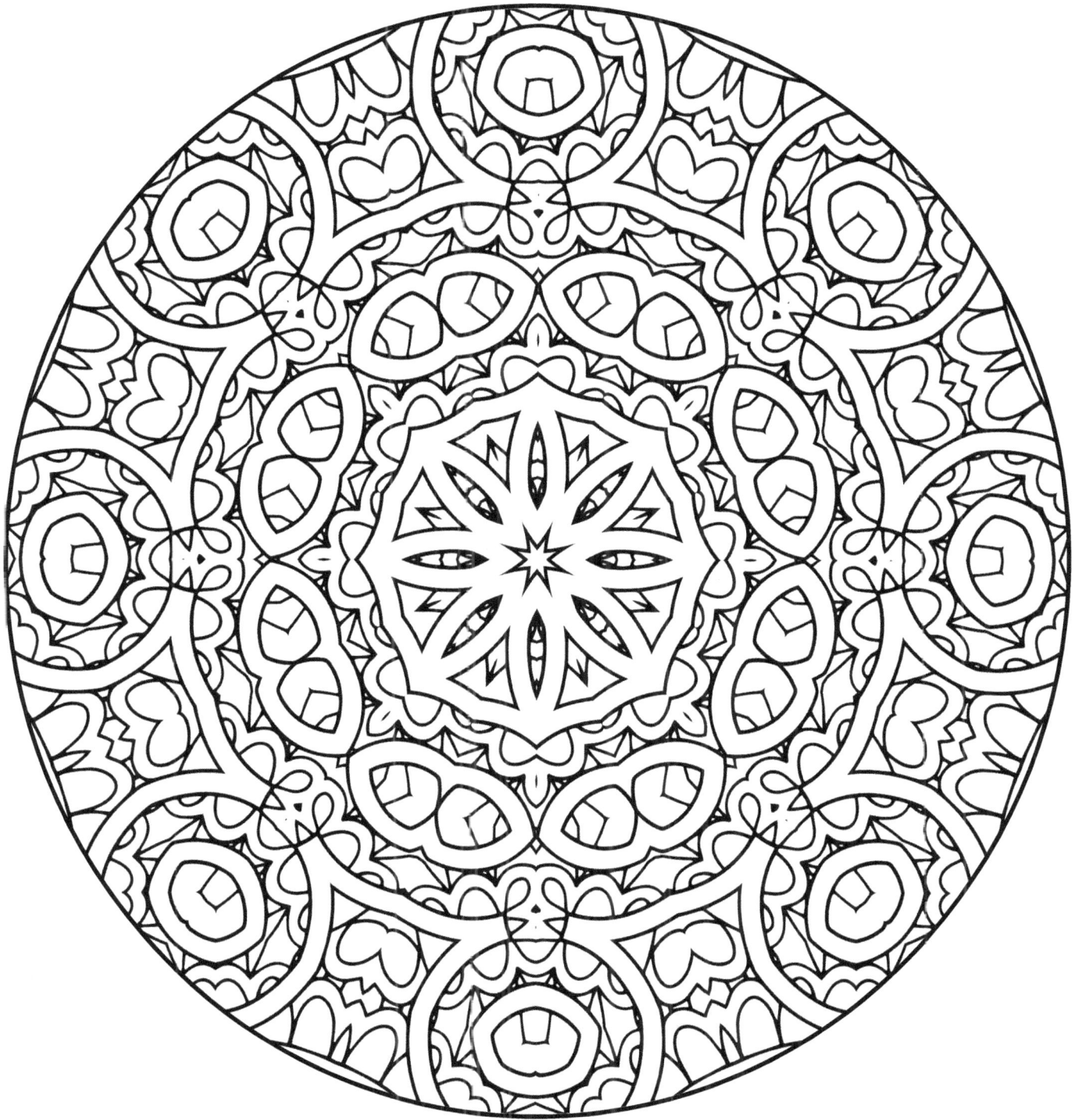

Date Completed: _____

Media Used:_____

_____

_____

Notes: _____

_____

_____

_____

_____

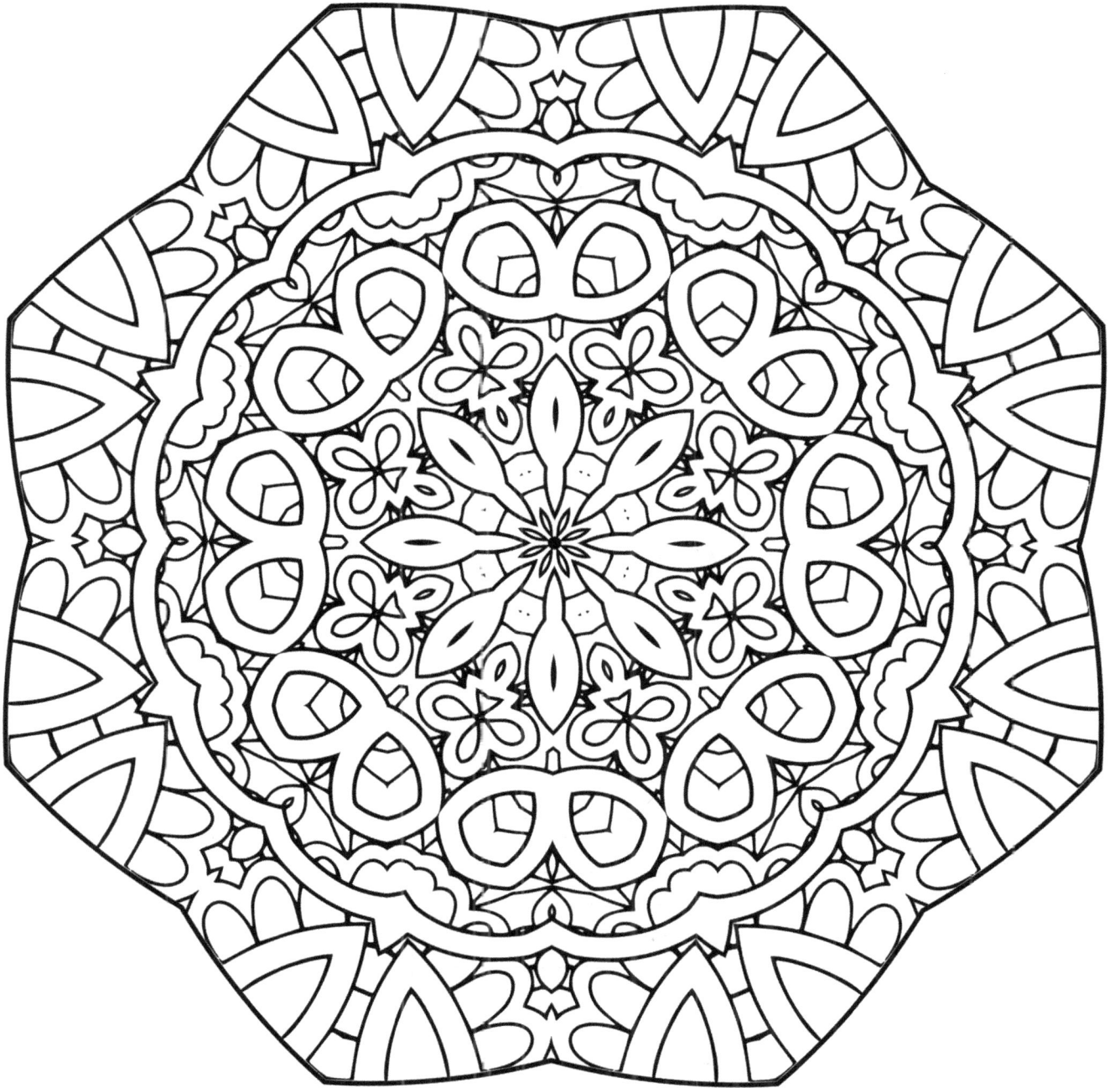

Date Completed: _____
Media Used:_____
_____
_____
Notes: _____
_____
_____
_____
_____
_____

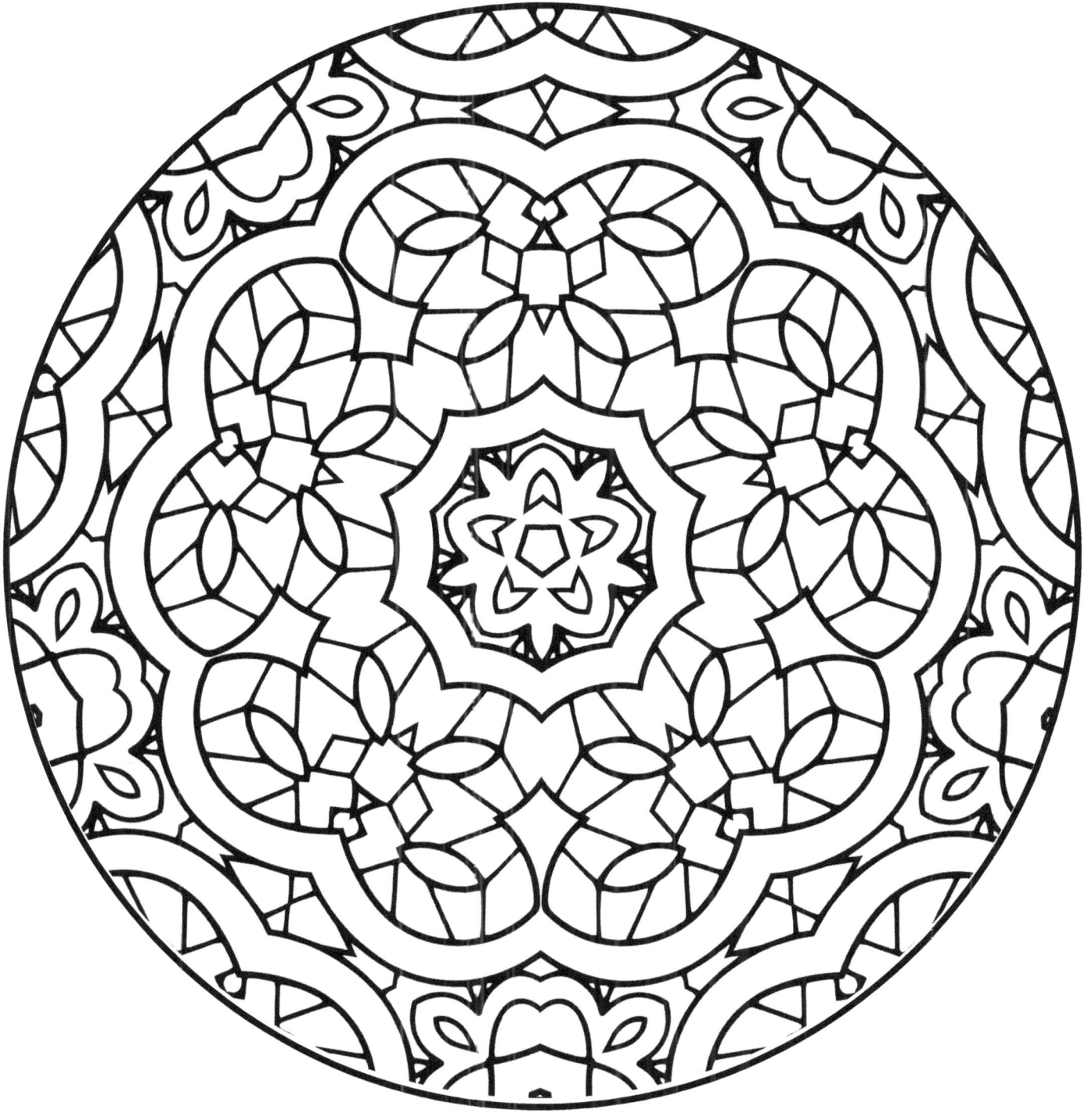

Date Completed: _____
Media Used:_____
_____
_____
Notes: __)_____
_____
_____
_____
_____

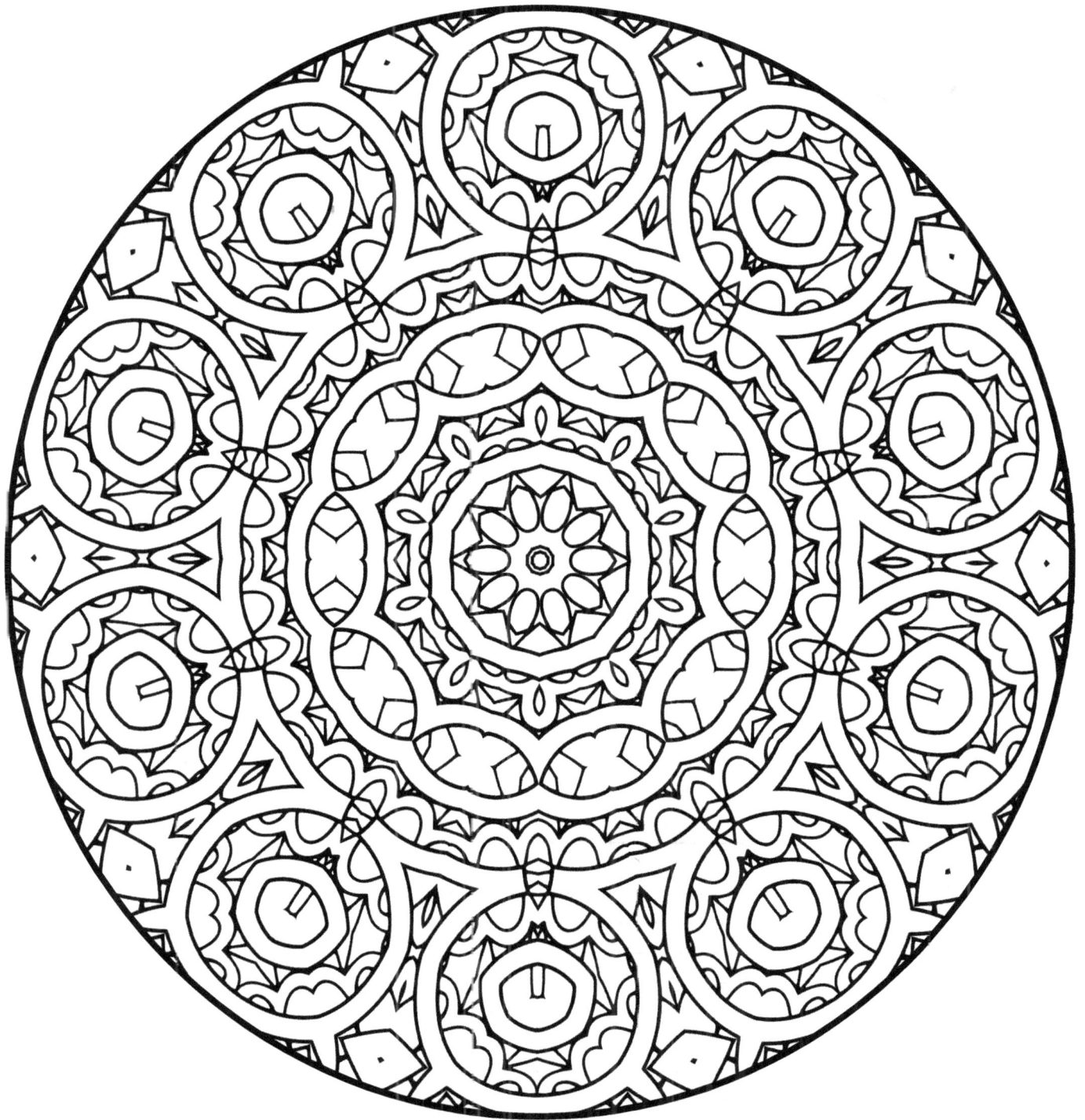

Date Completed: _____

Media Used:_____

_____

_____

Notes: _____

_____

_____

_____

_____

_____

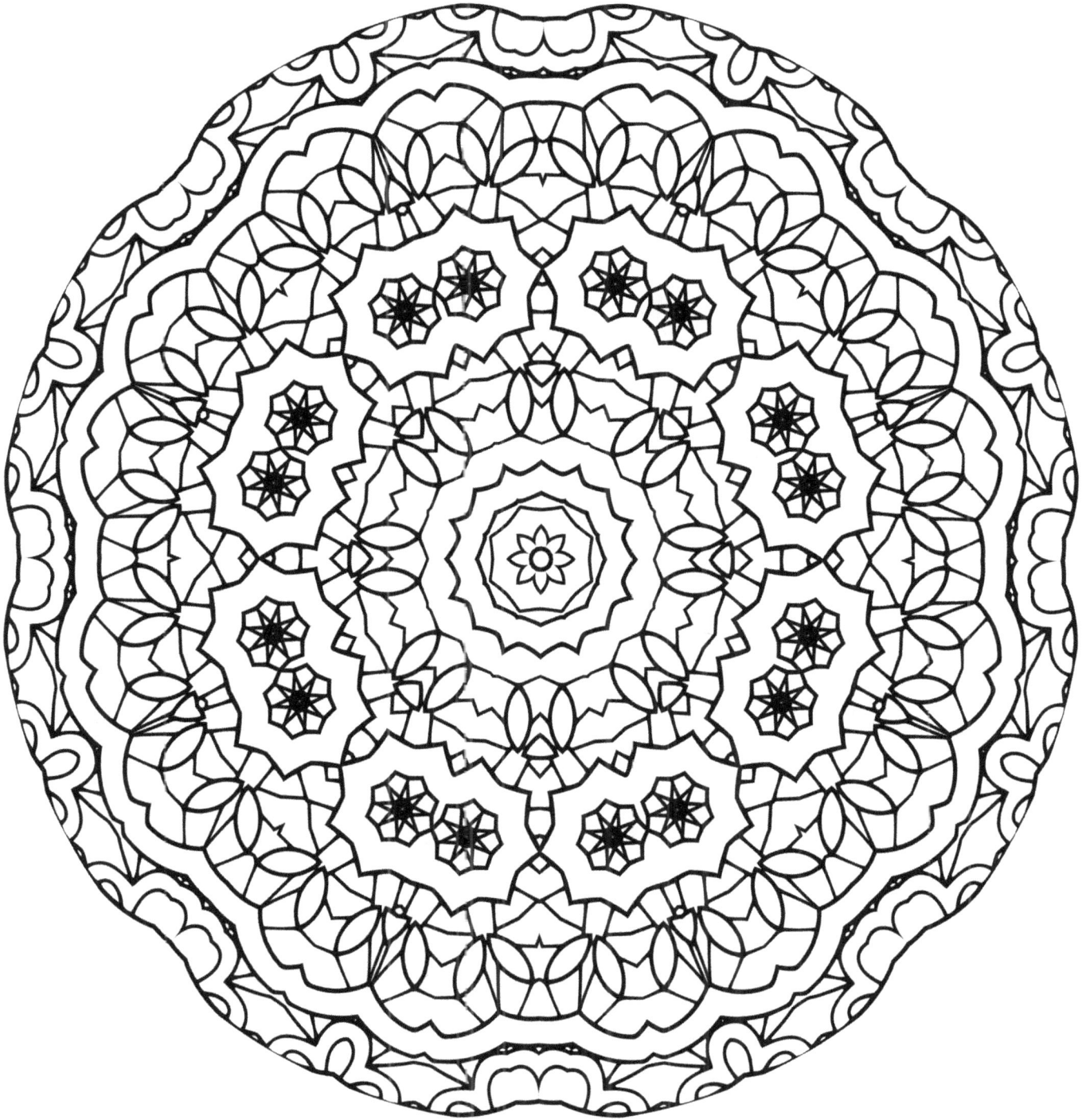

Date Completed: _____

Media Used:_____

_____

_____

Notes: _____

_____

_____

_____

_____

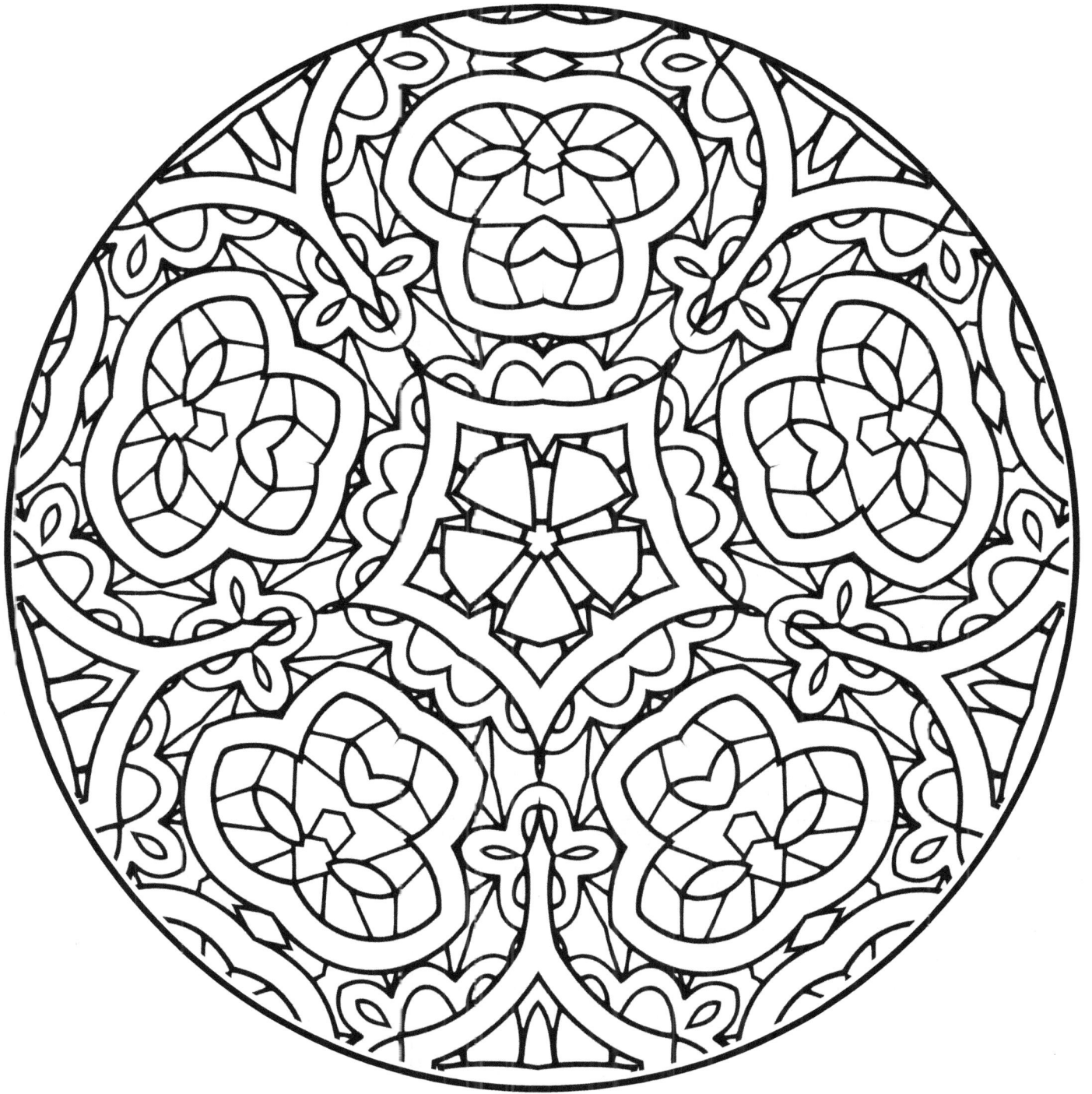

Date Completed: _____
Media Used:_____
_____
_____
Notes: _____
_____
_____
_____
_____

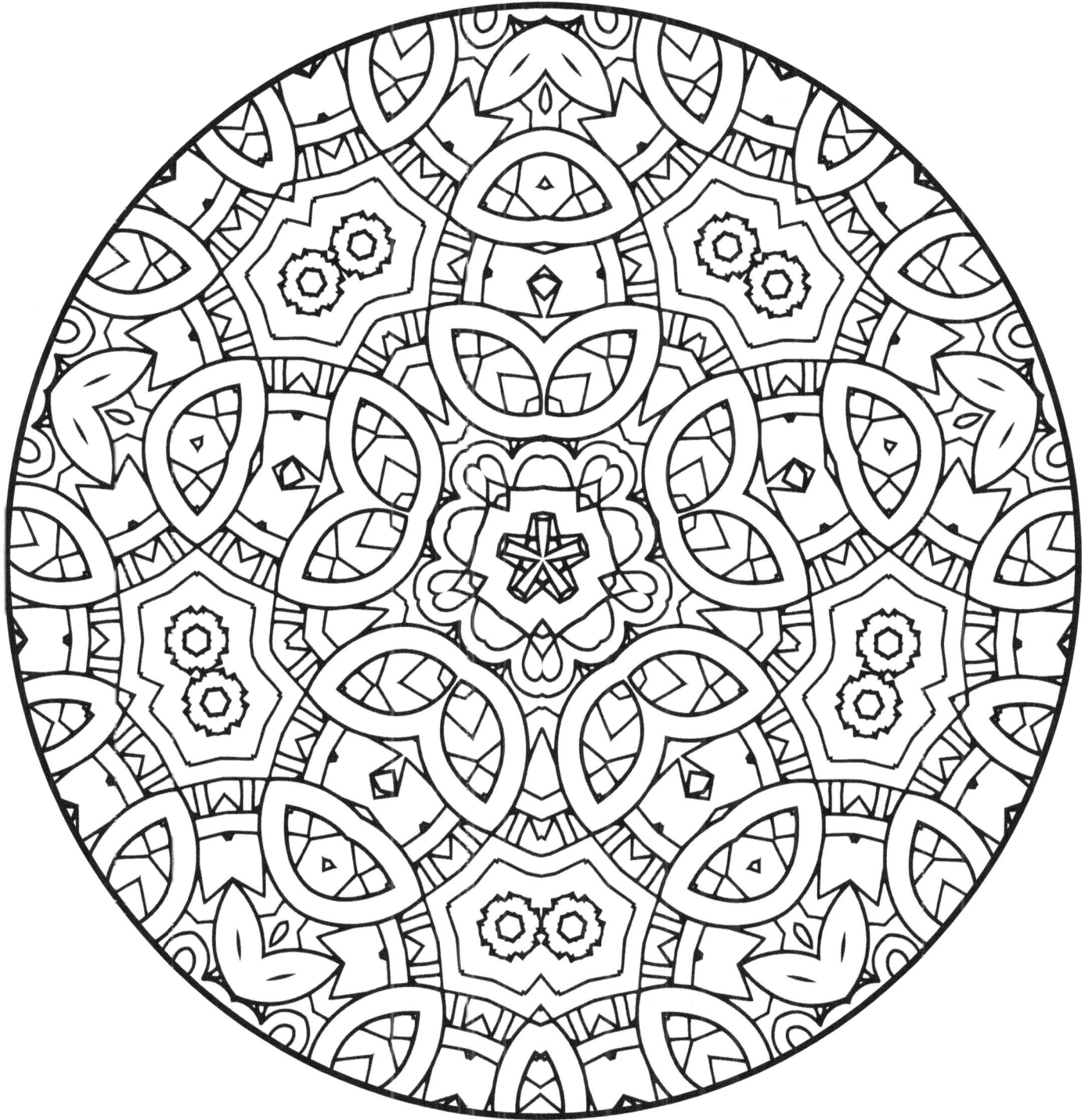

Date Completed: _____
Media Used:_____
_____
_____
Notes: _____
_____
_____
_____
_____

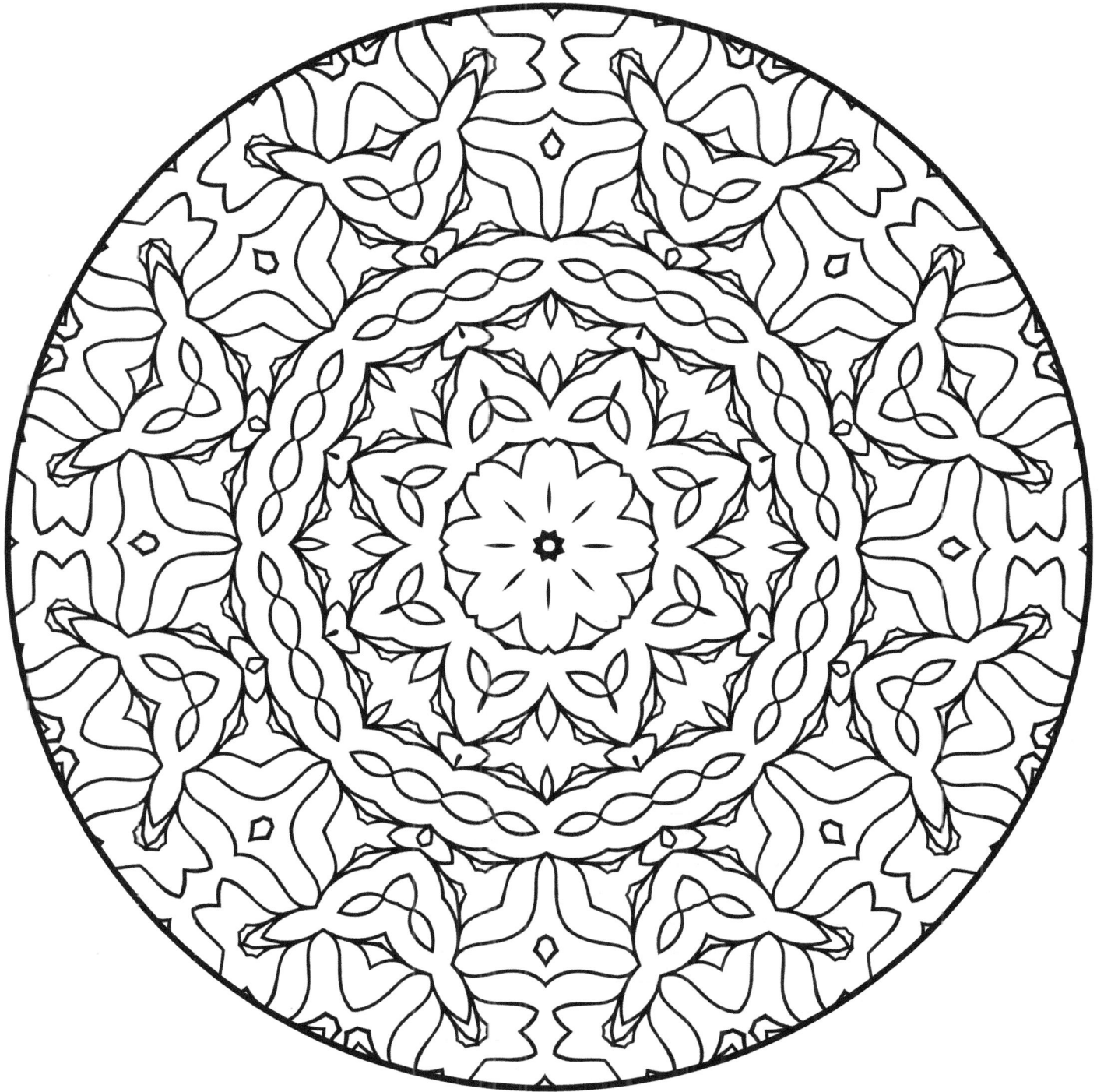

Date Completed: _____

Media Used:_____

_____

_____

Notes: _____

_____

_____

_____

_____

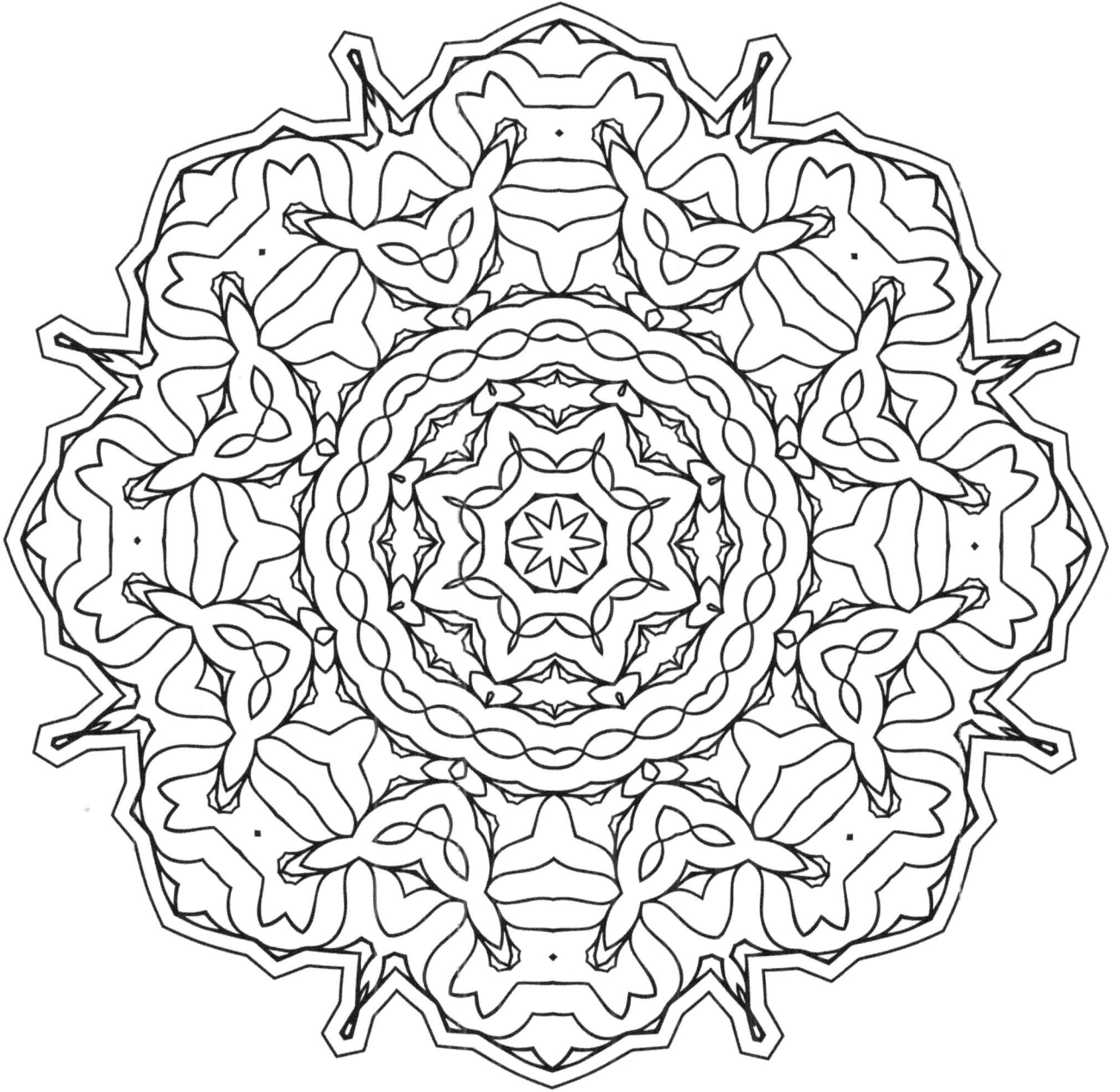

Date Completed: _____

Media Used:_____

_____

_____

Notes: _____

_____

_____

_____

_____

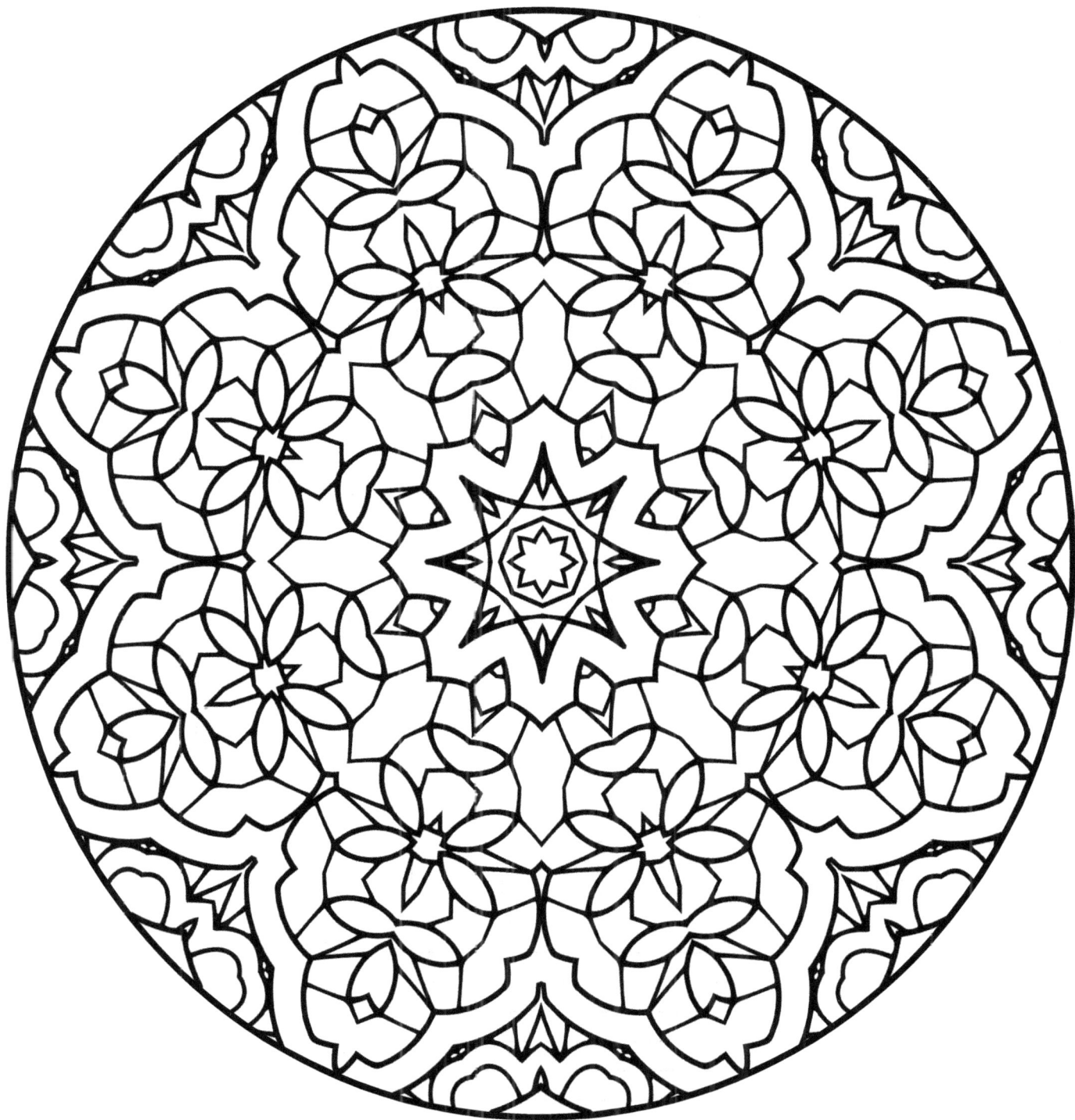

Date Completed: _____

Media Used:_____

_____

_____

Notes: _____

_____

_____

_____

_____

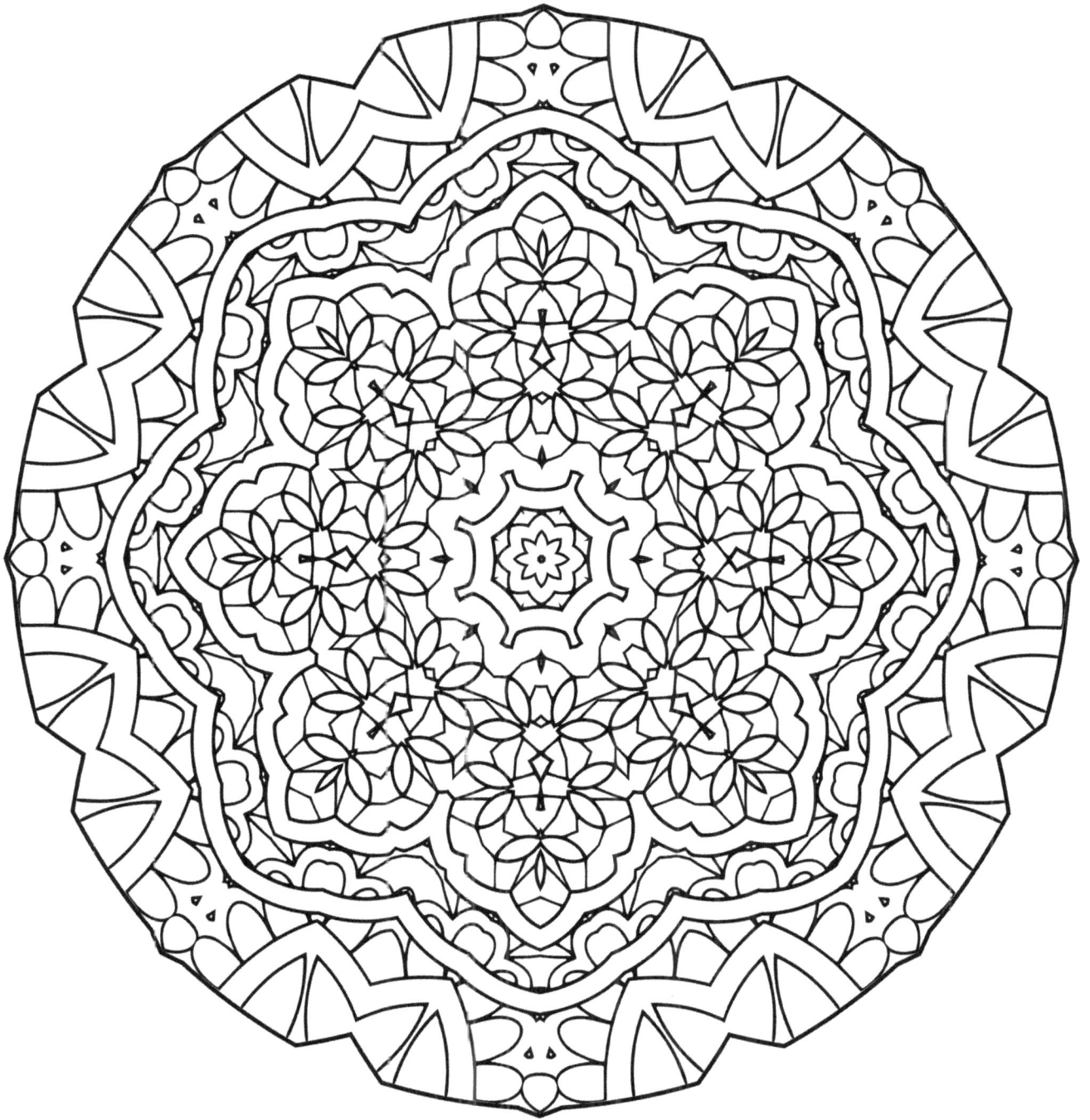

Date Completed: _____

Media Used: _____

_____

_____

Notes: _____

_____

_____

_____

_____

_____

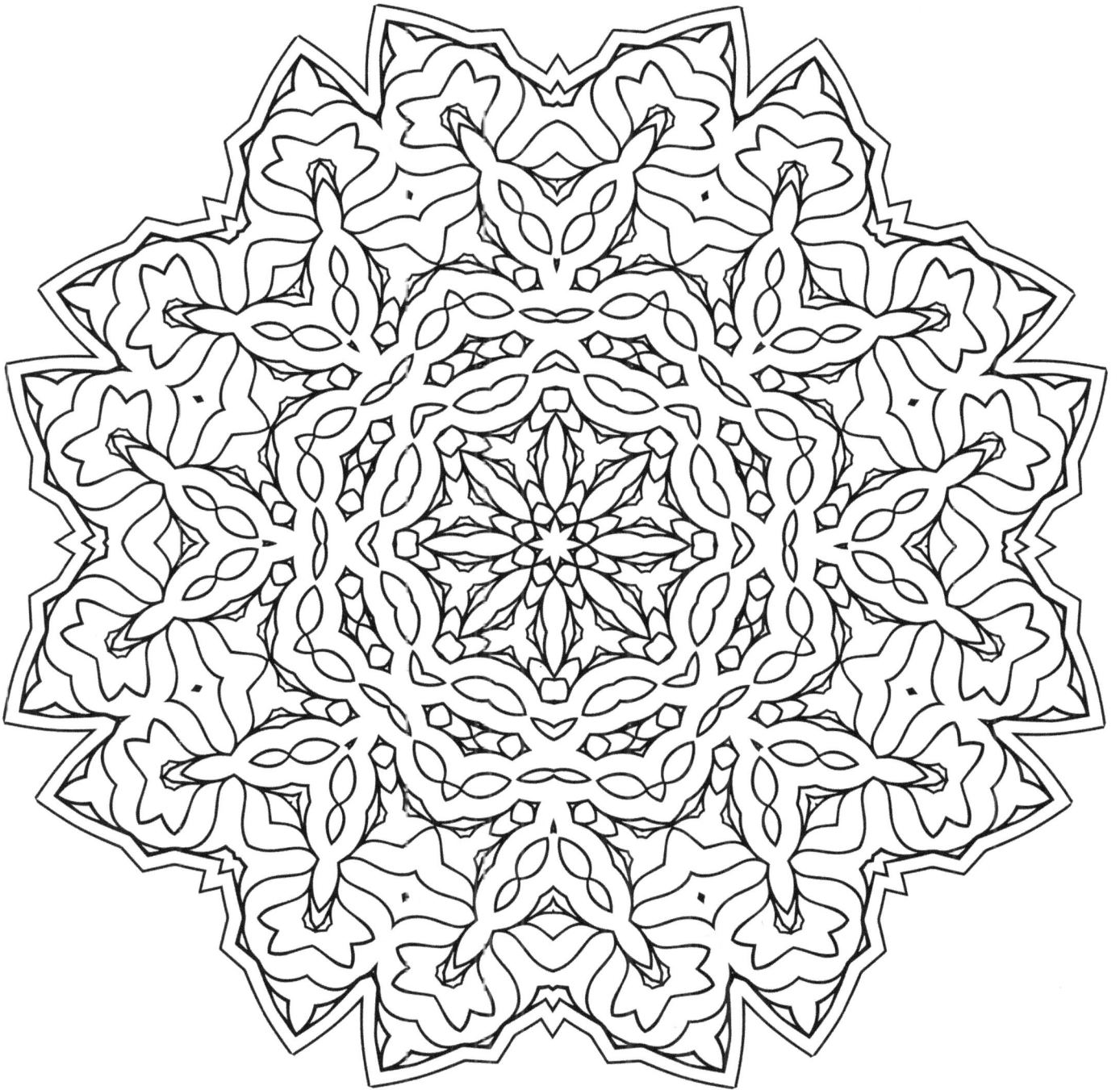

Date Completed: _____

Media Used:_____

_____

_____

Notes: _____

_____

_____

_____

_____

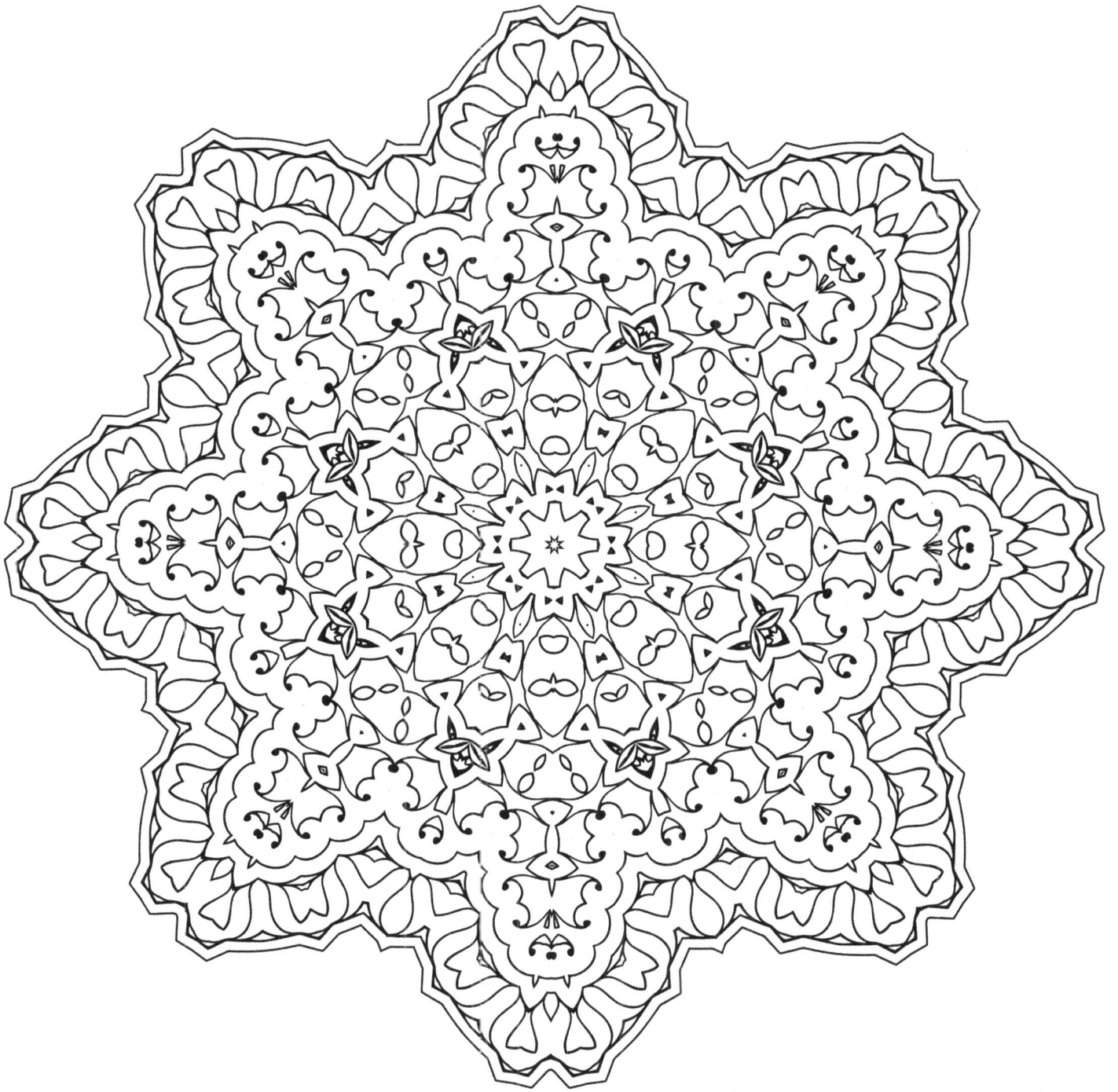

Date Completed: _____
Media Used:_____
_____
_____
Notes: _____
_____
_____
_____
_____

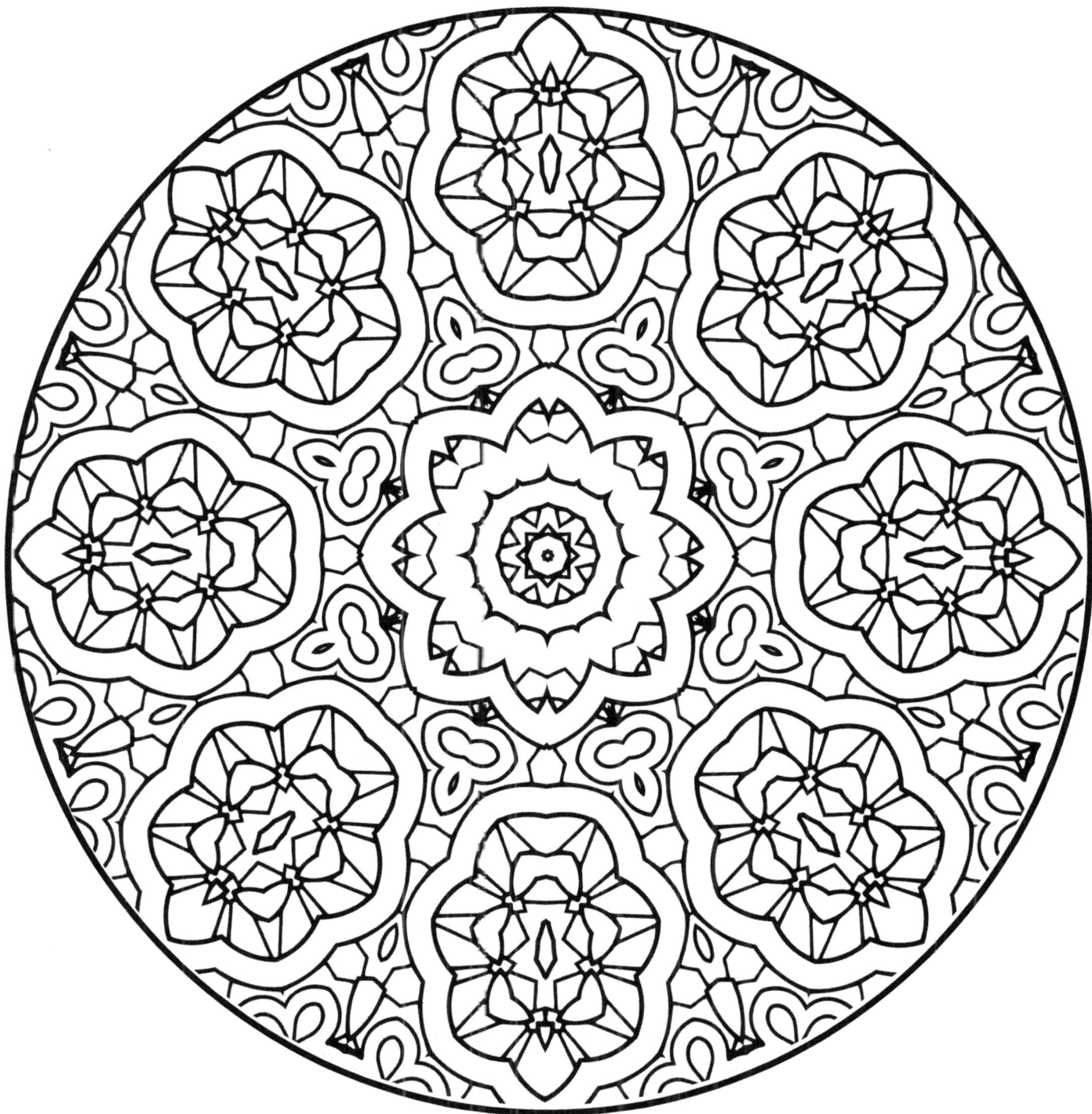

Date Completed: _____
Media Used:_____
_____
_____
Notes: _____
_____
_____
_____
_____

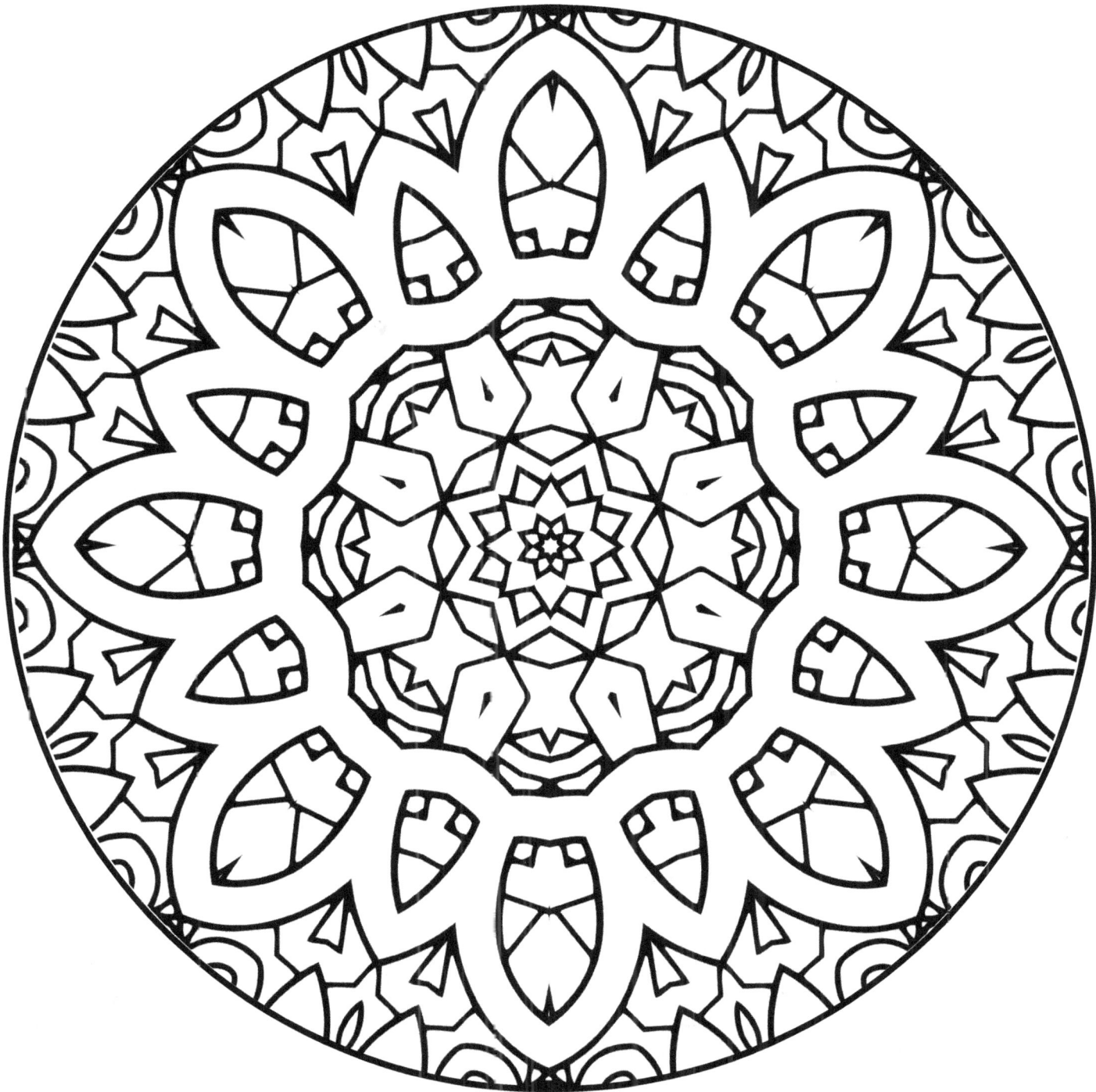

Date Completed: _____

Media Used:_____

_____

_____

Notes: _____

_____

_____

_____

_____

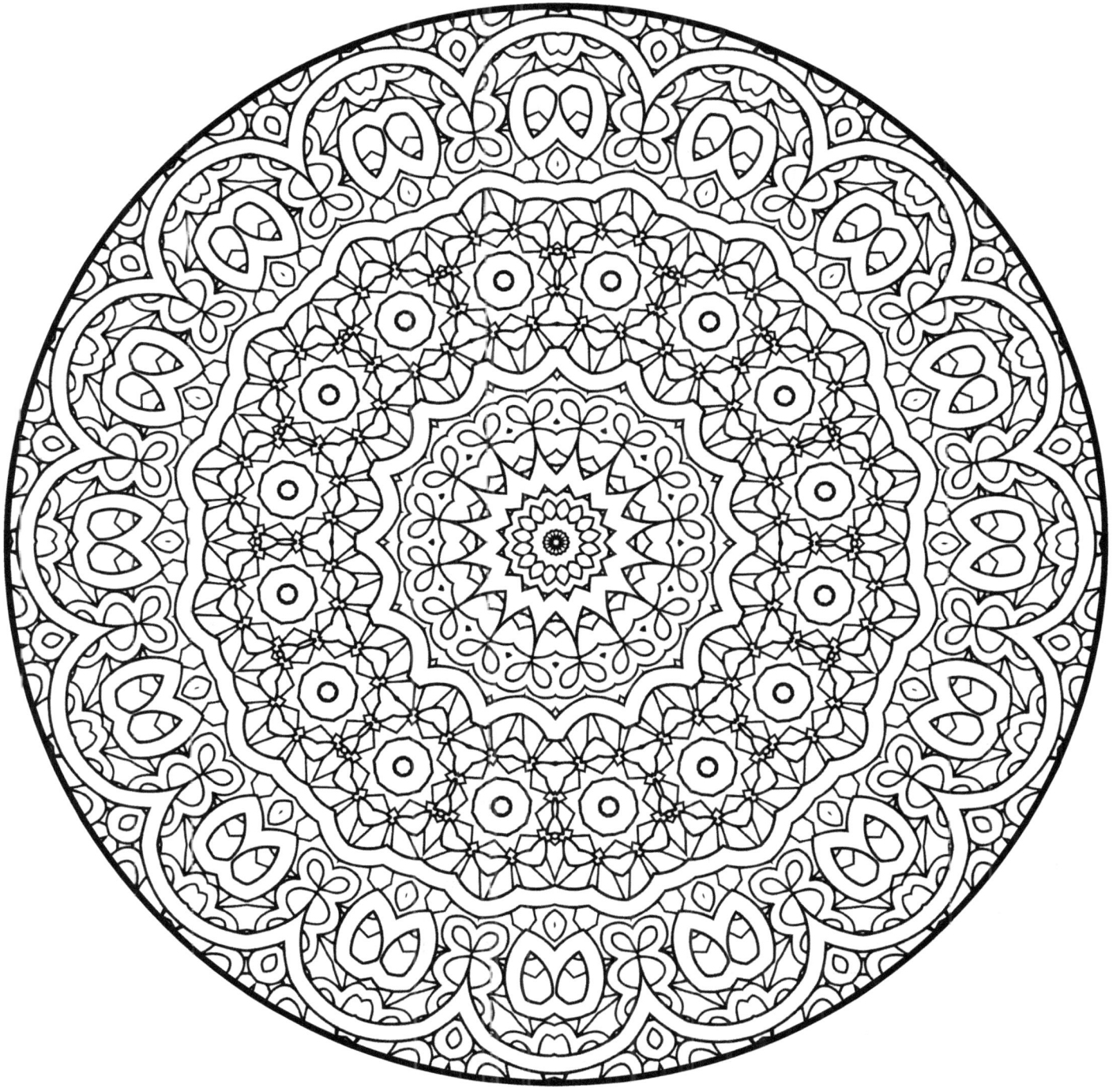

Date Completed: _____

Media Used:_____

_____

_____

Notes: _____

_____

_____

_____

_____

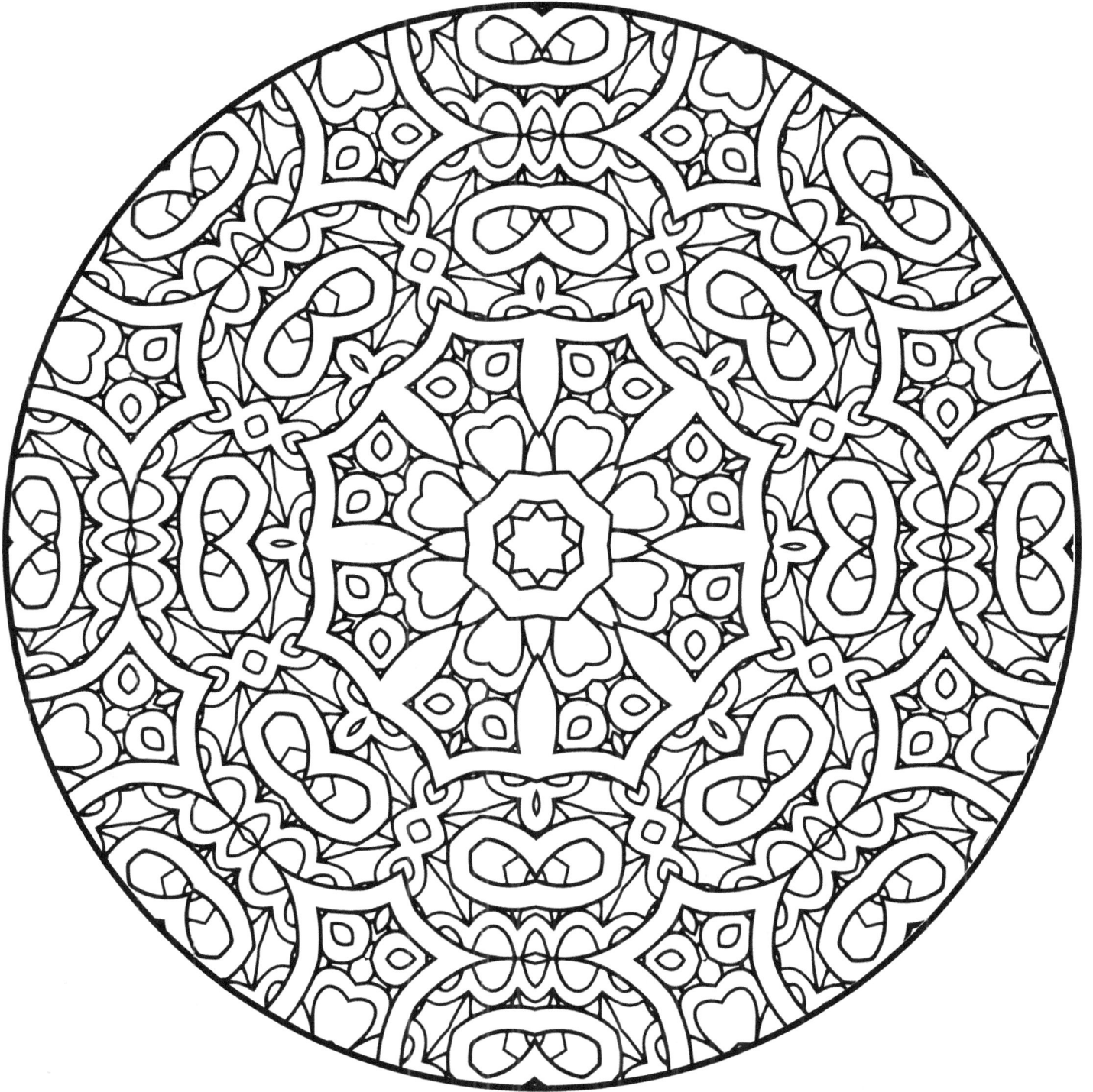

Date Completed: _____

Media Used:_____

_____

_____

Notes: _____

_____

_____

_____

_____

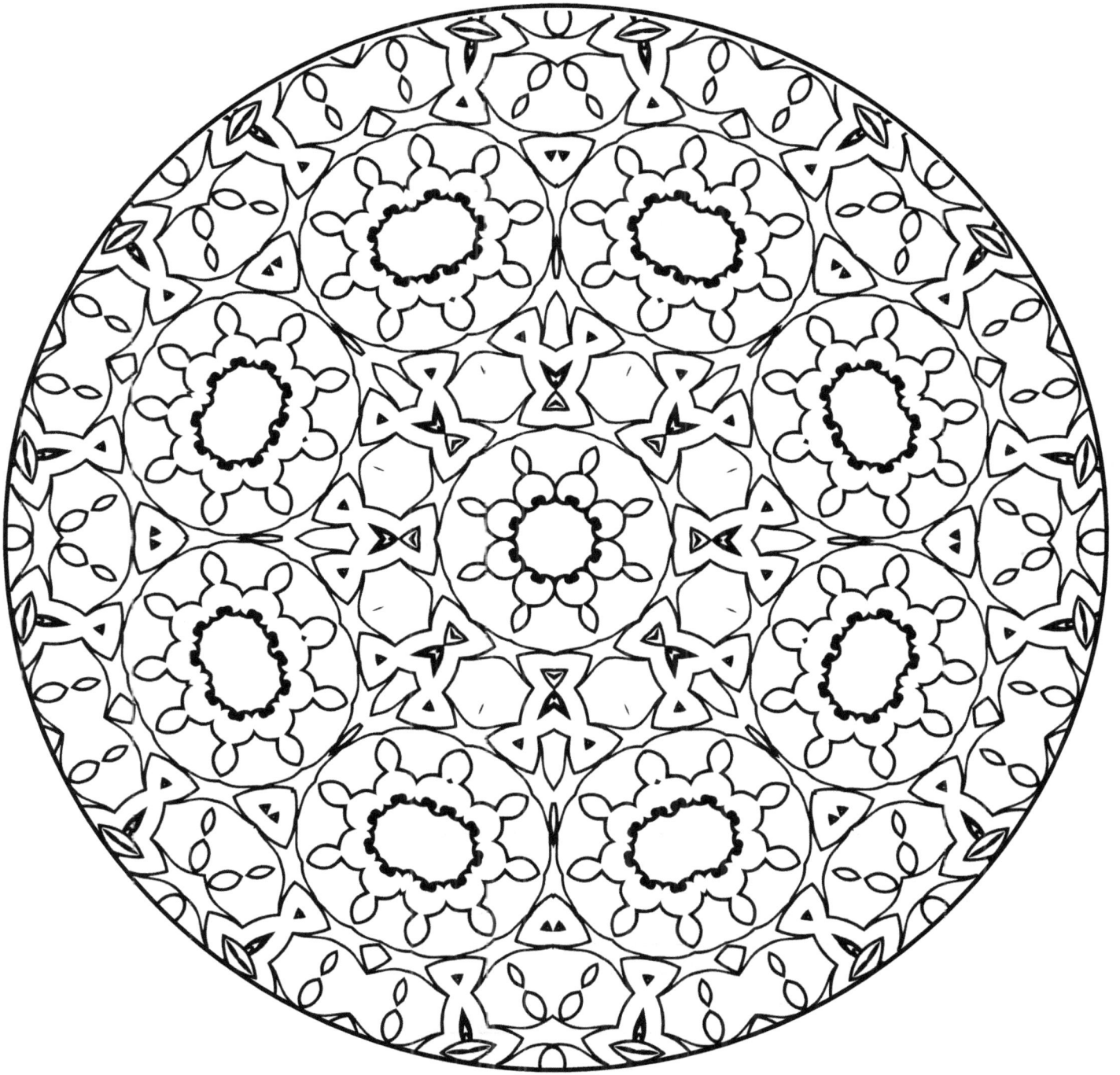

Date Completed: _____
Media Used:_____
_____
_____
Notes: _____
_____
_____
_____
_____
_____

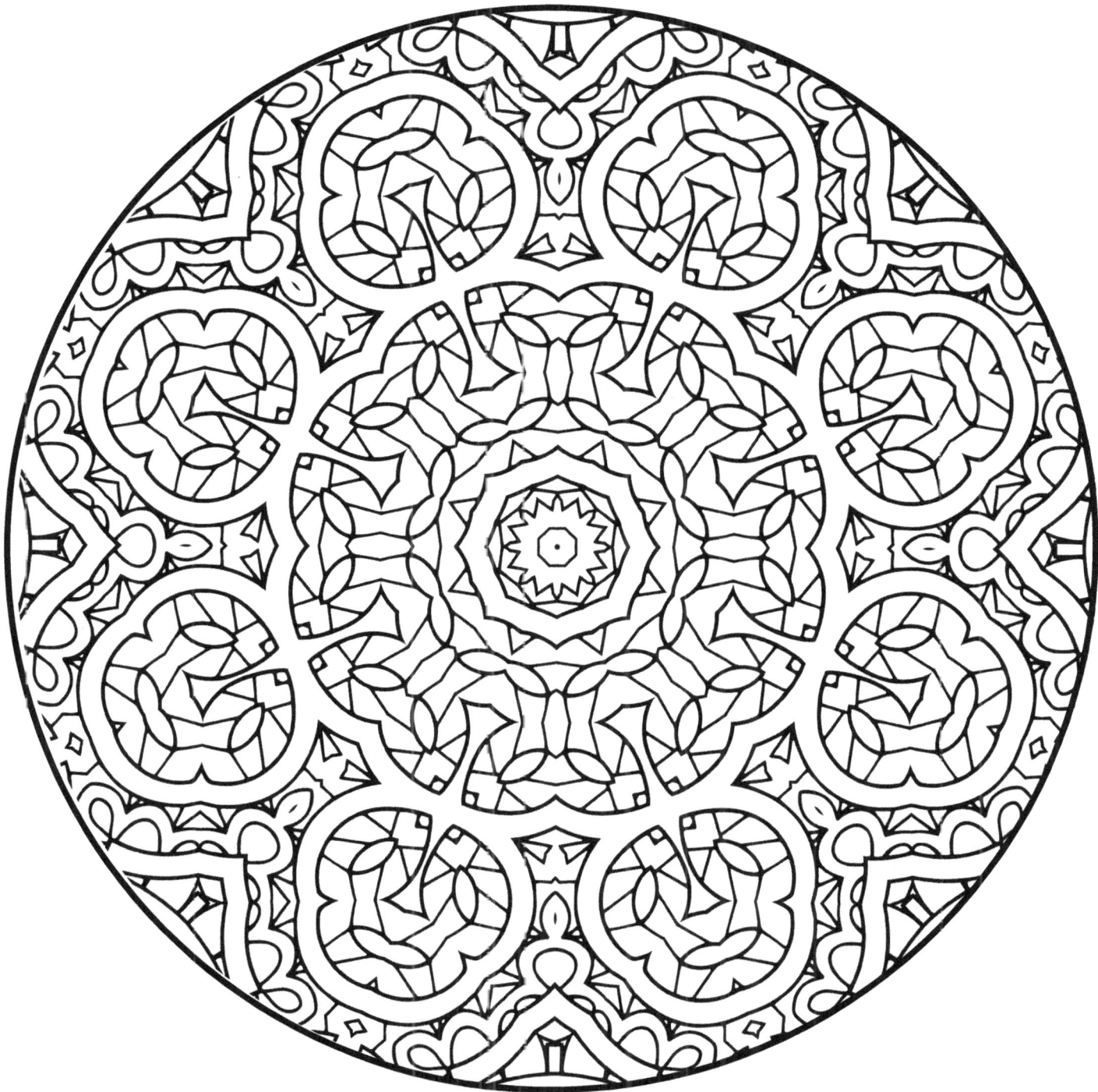

Date Completed: _____

Media Used:_____

_____

_____

Notes: _____

_____

_____

_____

_____

_____

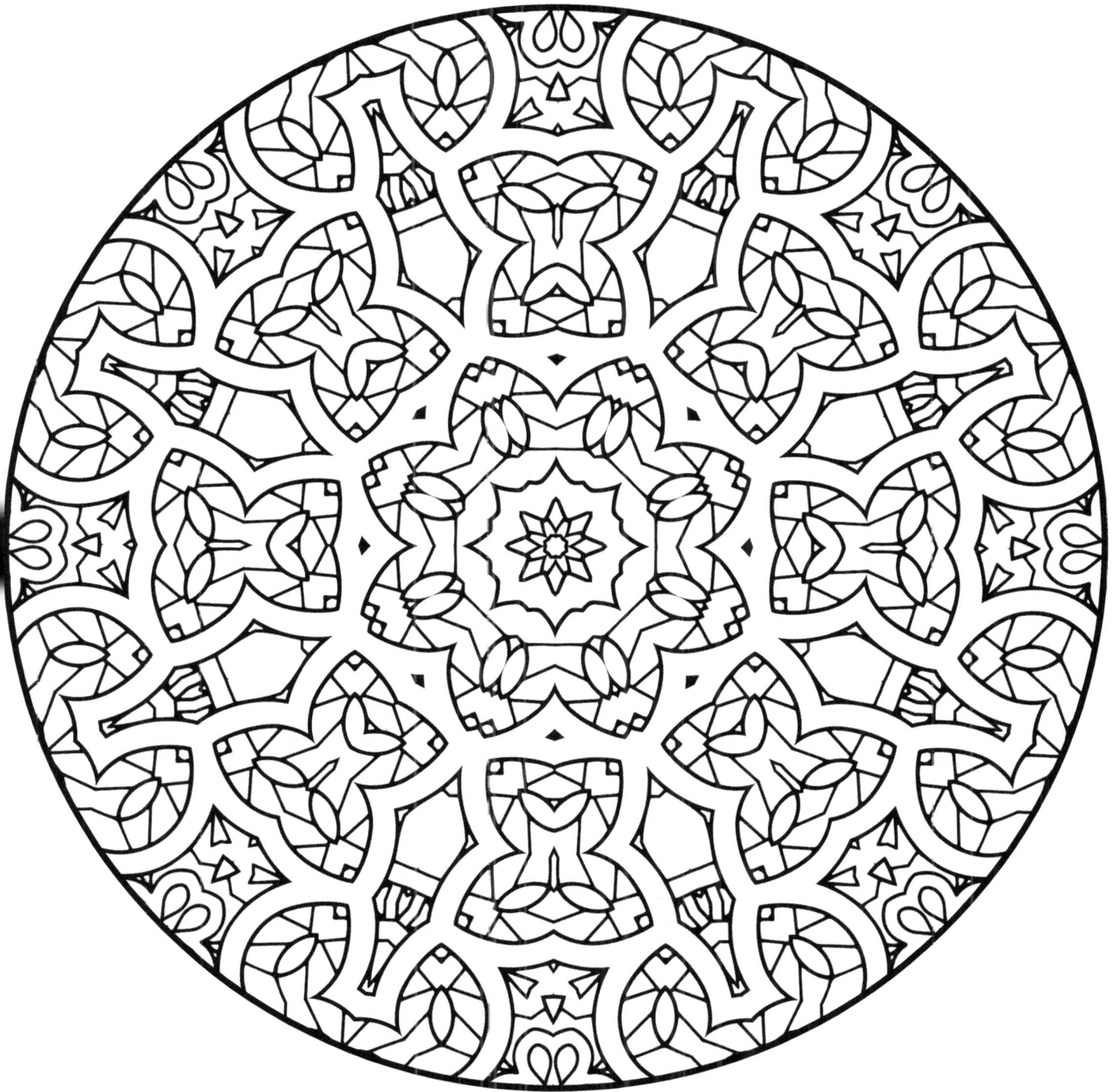

Date Completed: _____
Media Used:_____
_____
_____
Notes: _____
_____
_____
_____
_____

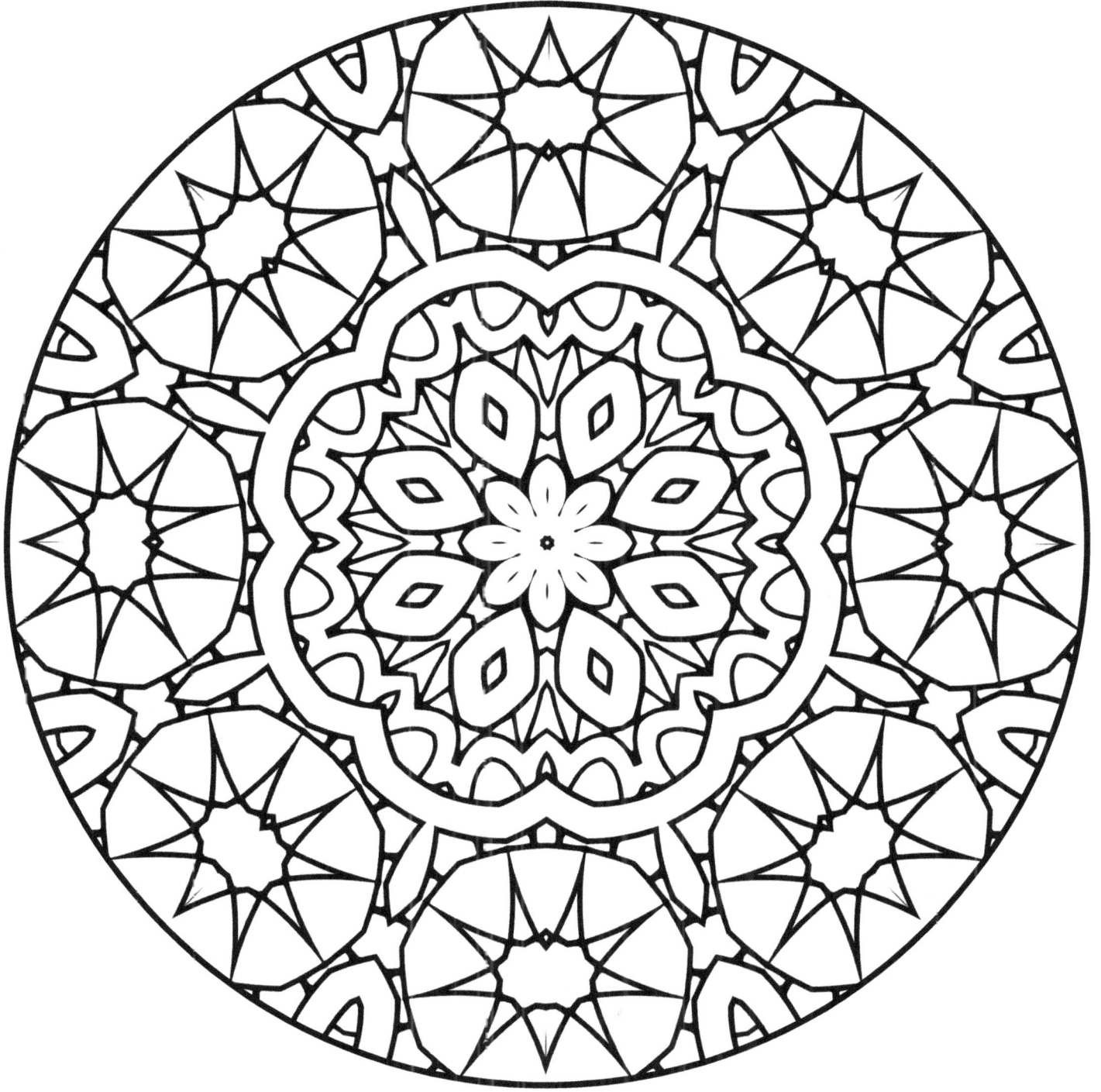

Date Completed: _____
Media Used:_____
_____
_____
Notes: _____
_____
_____
_____
_____

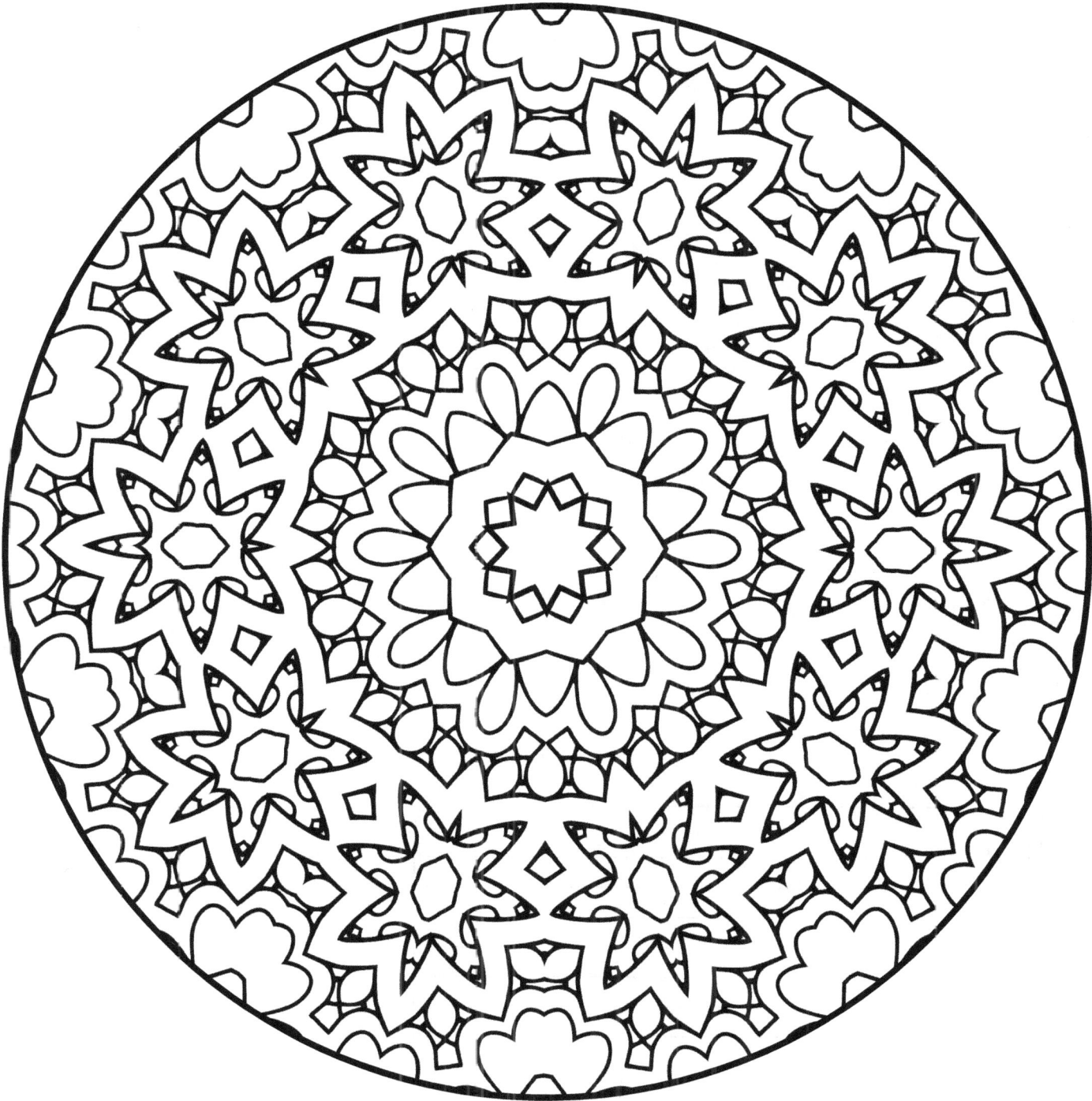

Date Completed: _____

Media Used:_____

_____

_____

Notes: _____

_____

_____

_____

_____

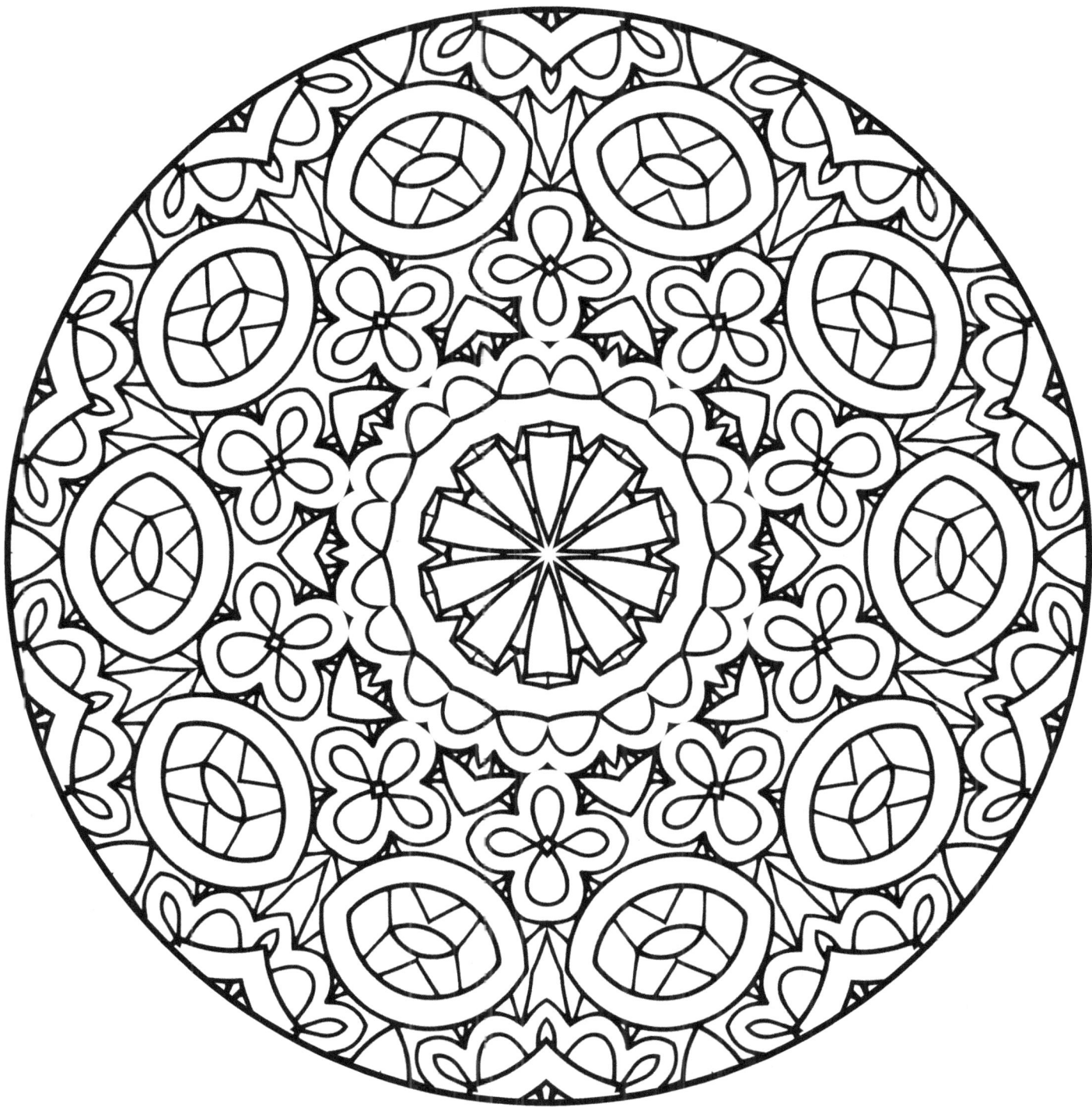

Date Completed: _____

Media Used:_____

_____

_____

Notes: _____

_____

_____

_____

_____

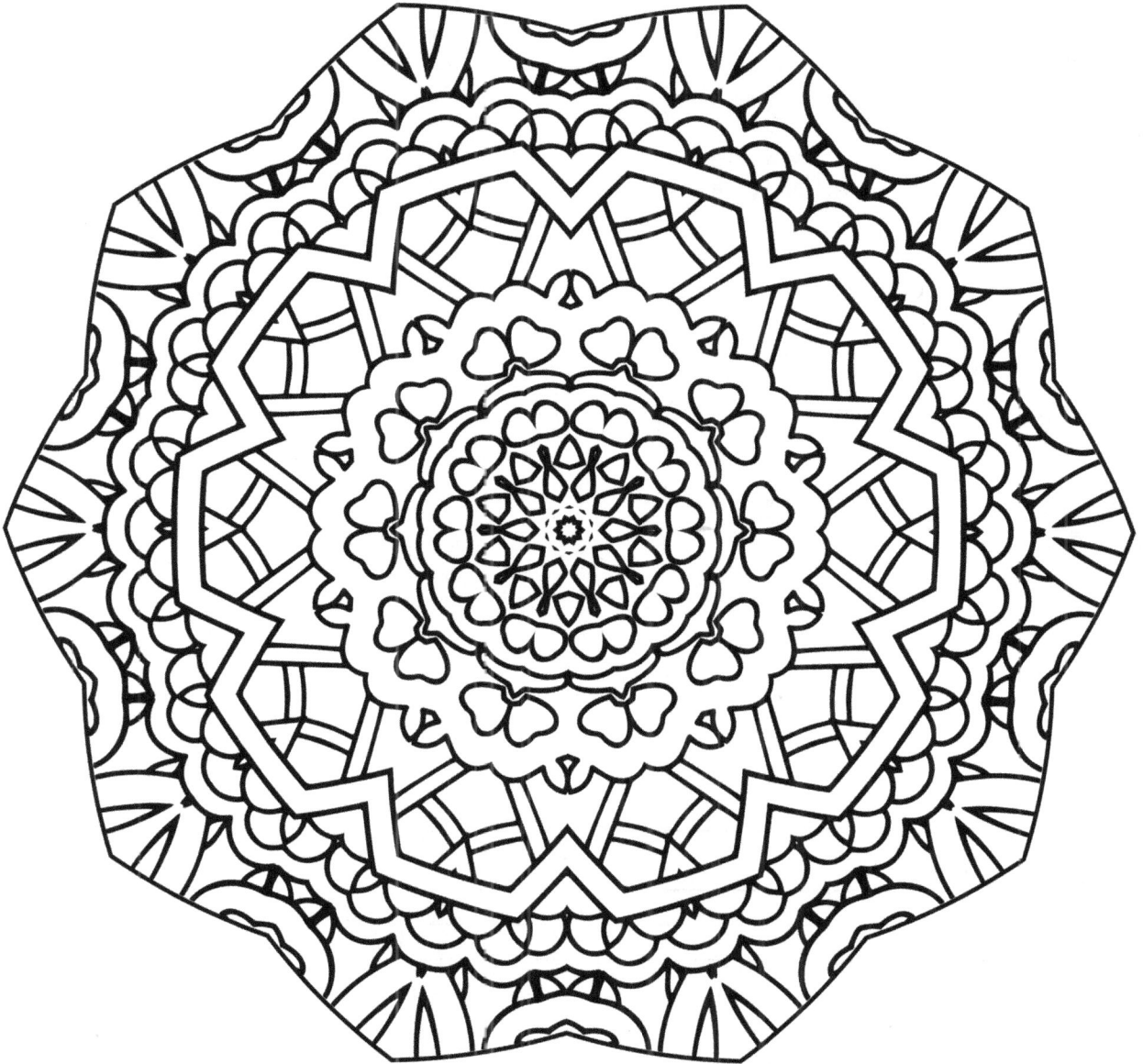

Date Completed: _____

Media Used:_____

_____

_____

Notes: _____

_____

_____

_____

_____

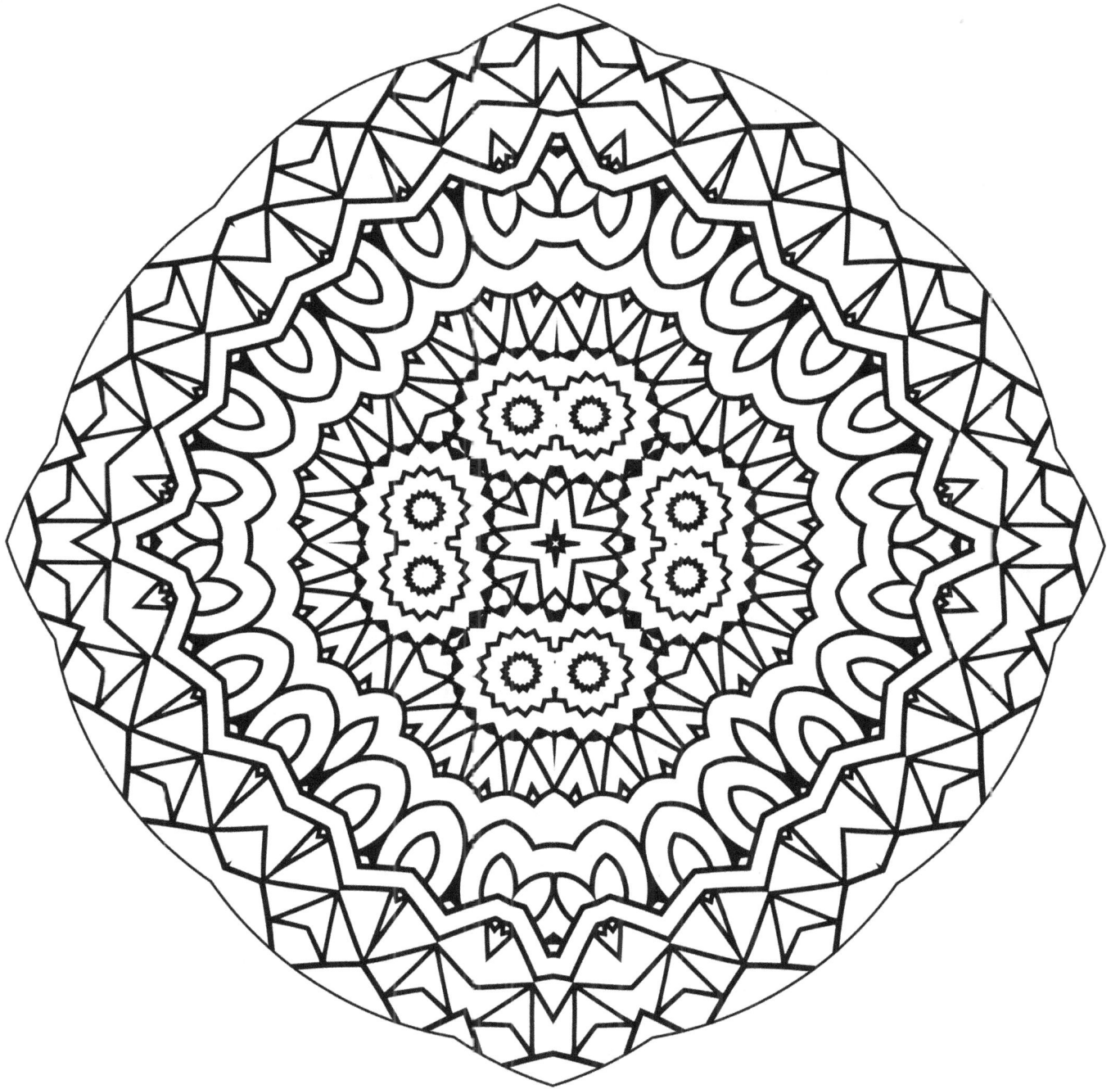

Date Completed: _____
Media Used:_____
_____
_____
Notes: _____
_____
_____
_____
_____
_____

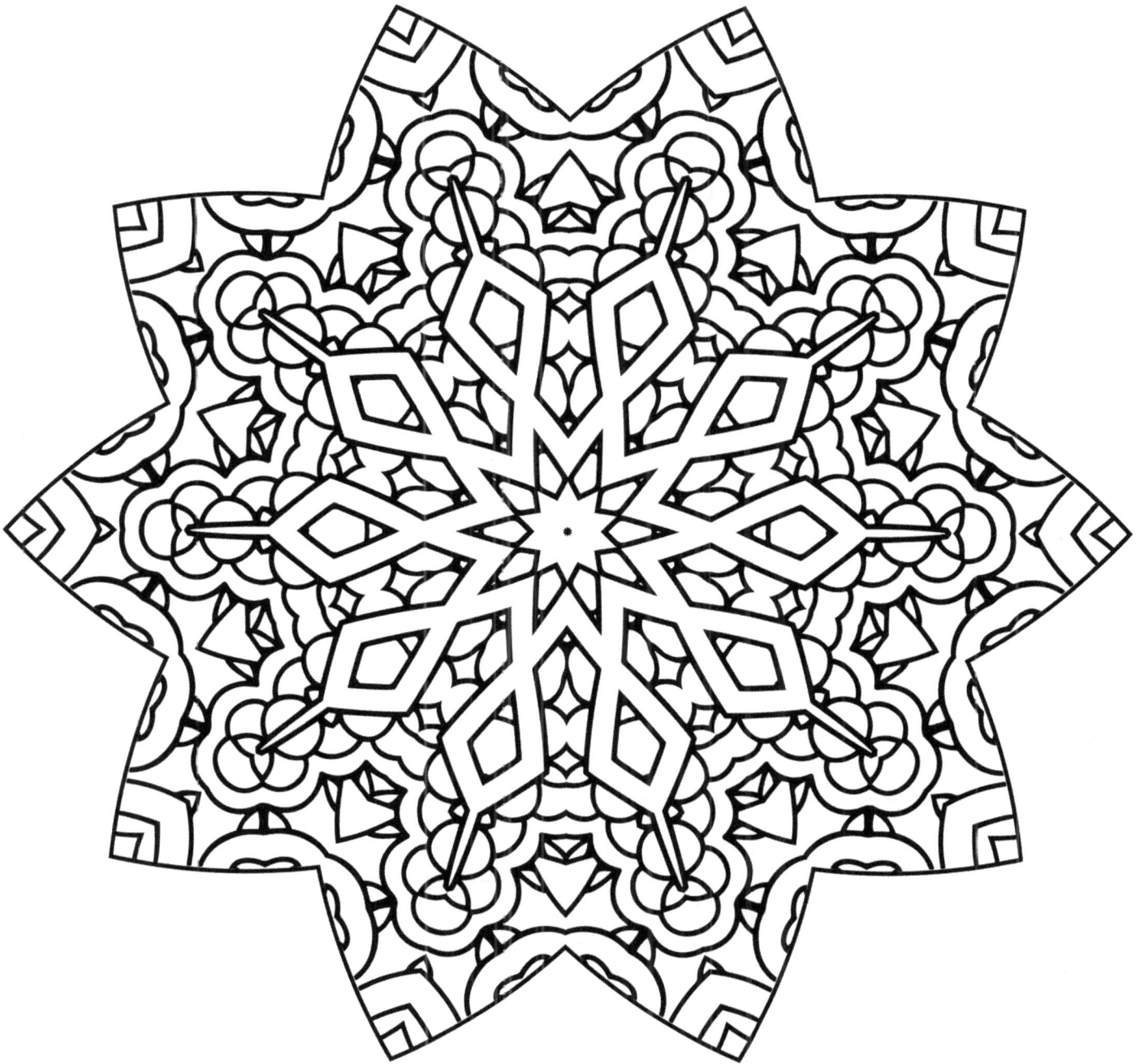

Date Completed: _____

Media Used:_____

_____

_____

Notes: _____

_____

_____

_____

_____

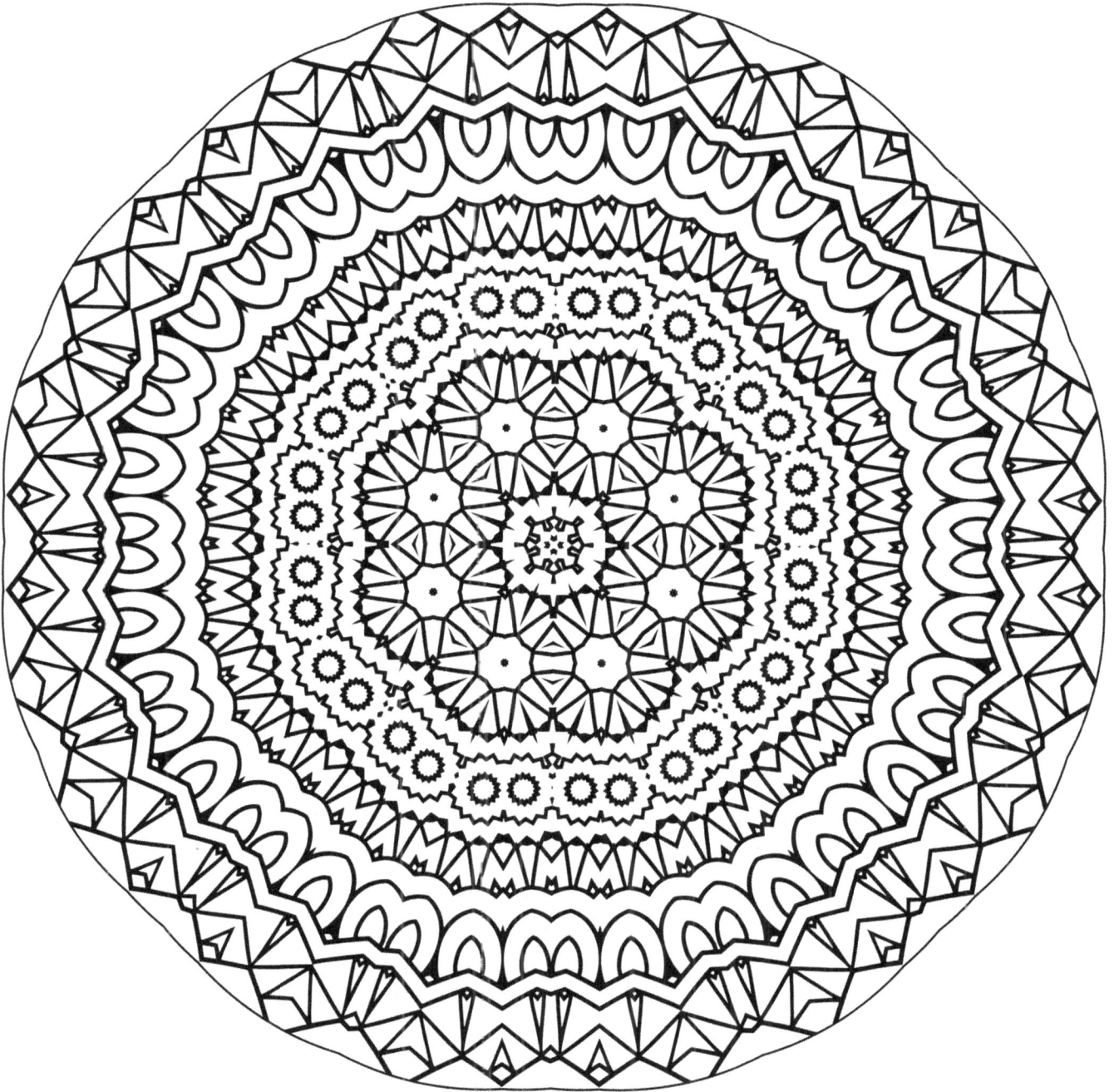

Date Completed: _____

Media Used: _____

_____

_____

Notes: _____

_____

_____

_____

_____

_____

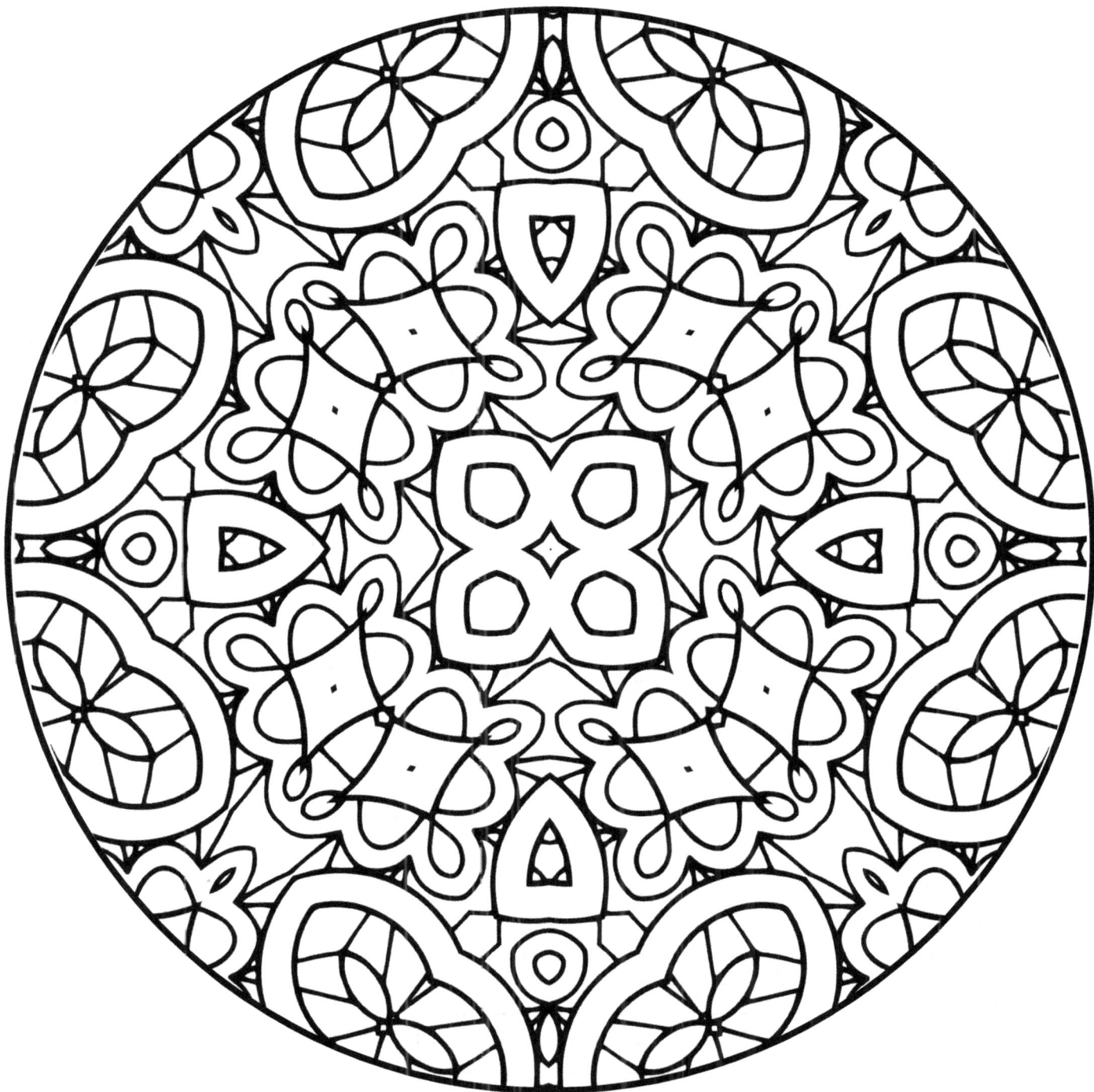

Date Completed: _____
Media Used:_____
_____
_____
Notes: _____
_____
_____
_____
_____

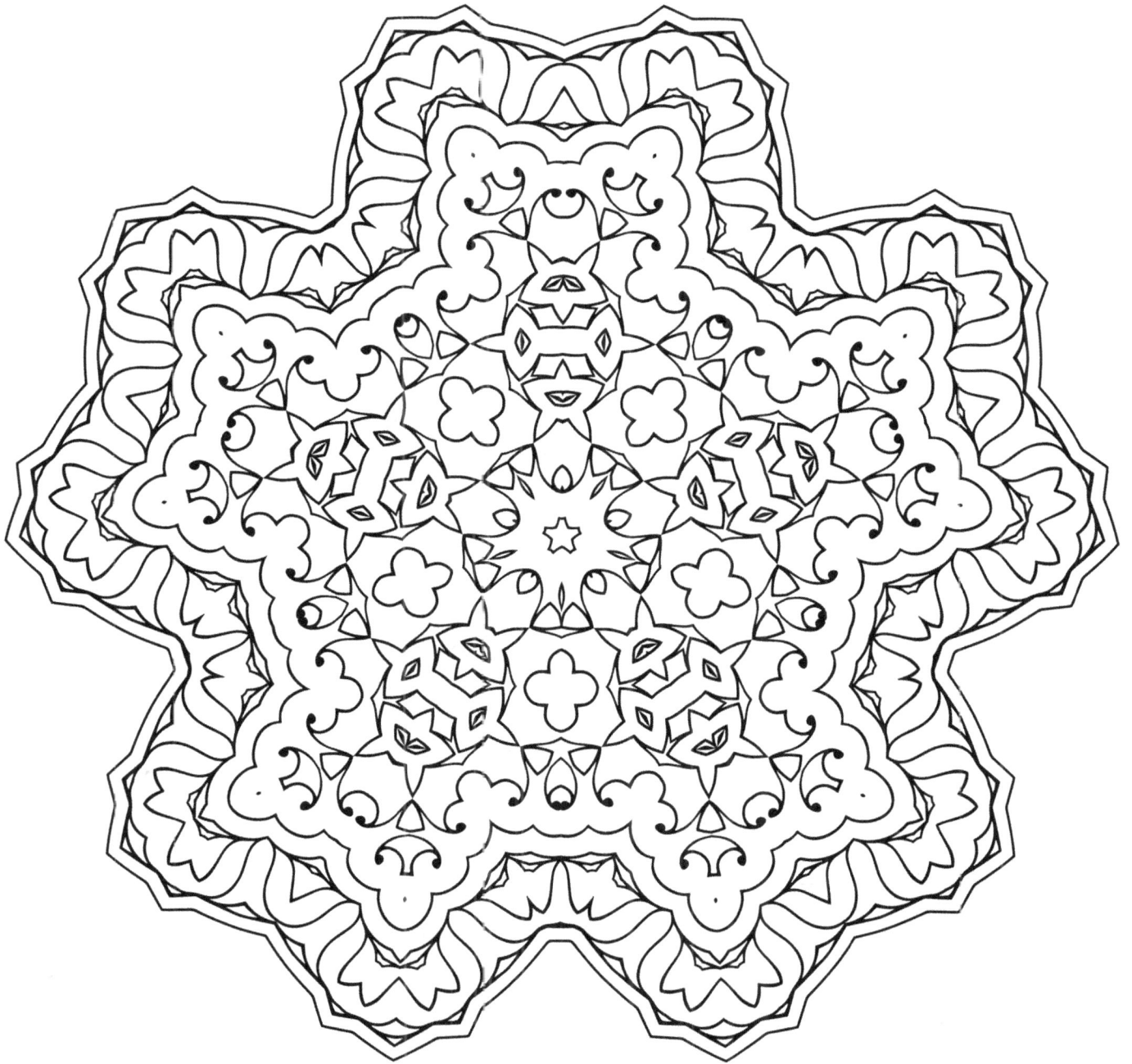

Date Completed: _____

Media Used:_____

_____

_____

Notes: _____

_____

_____

_____

_____

_____

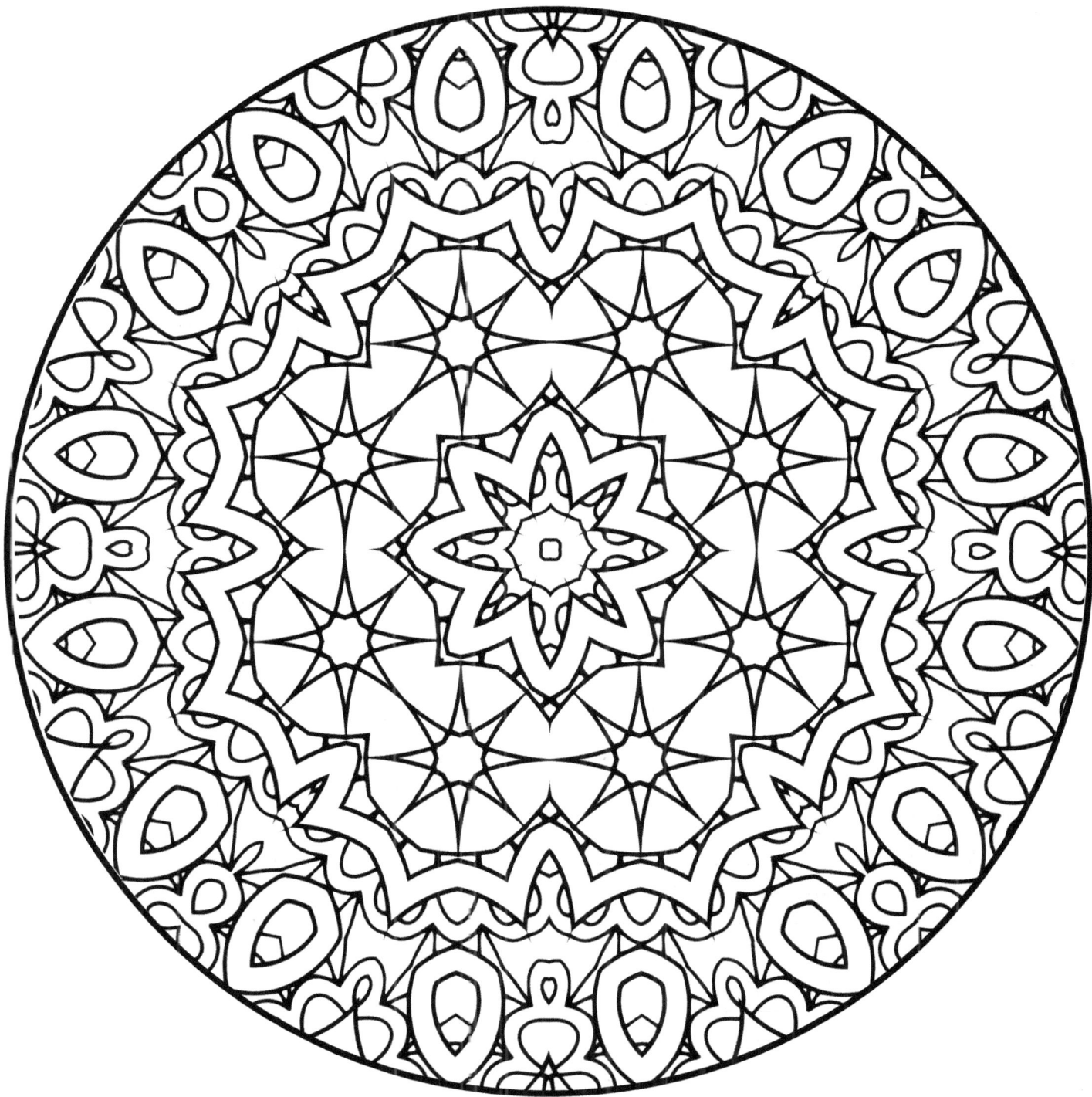

Date Completed: _____
Media Used:_____
_____
_____
Notes: _____
_____
_____
_____
_____

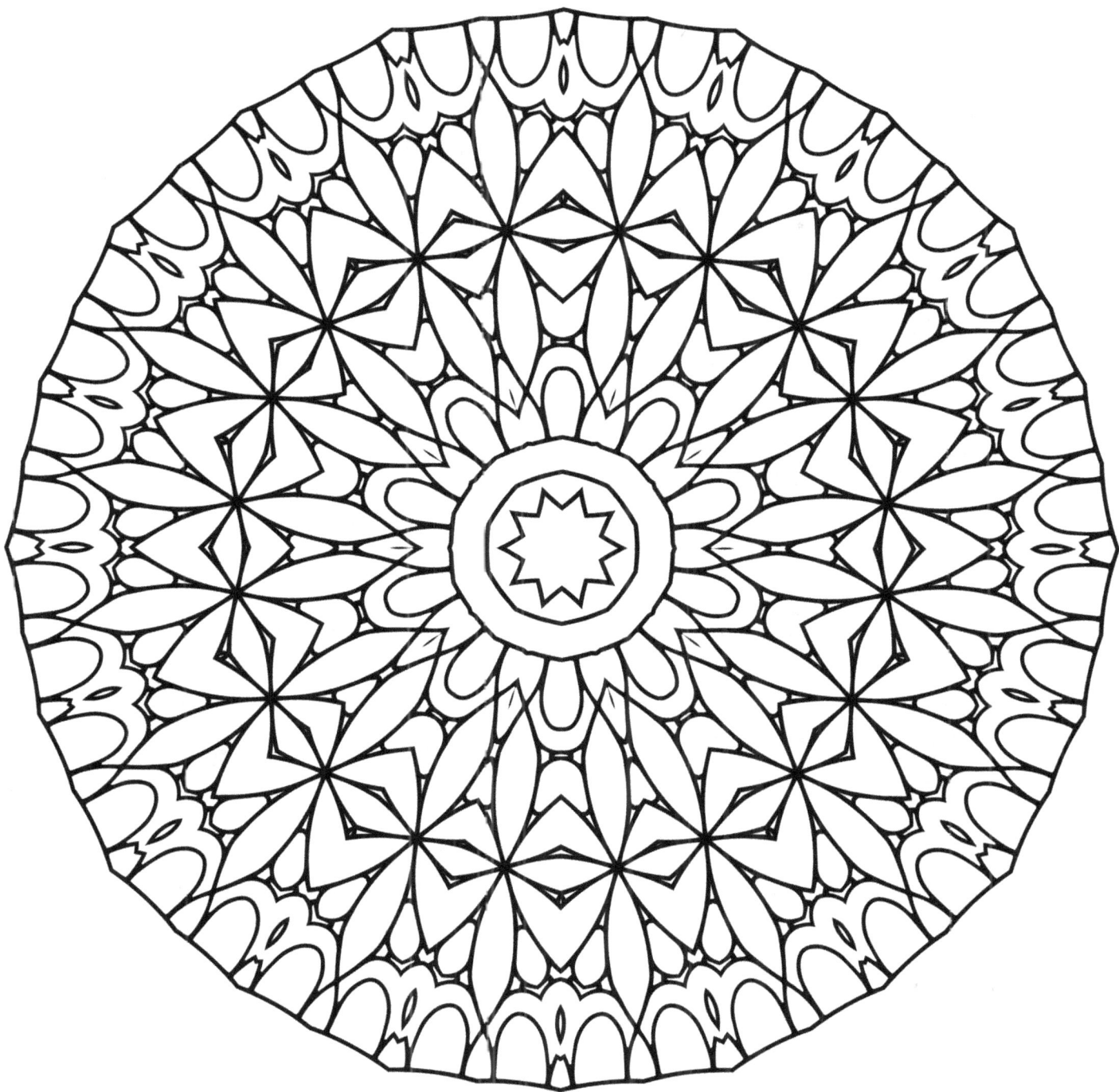

Date Completed: _____
Media Used:_____
_____
_____
Notes: _____
_____
_____
_____
_____
_____

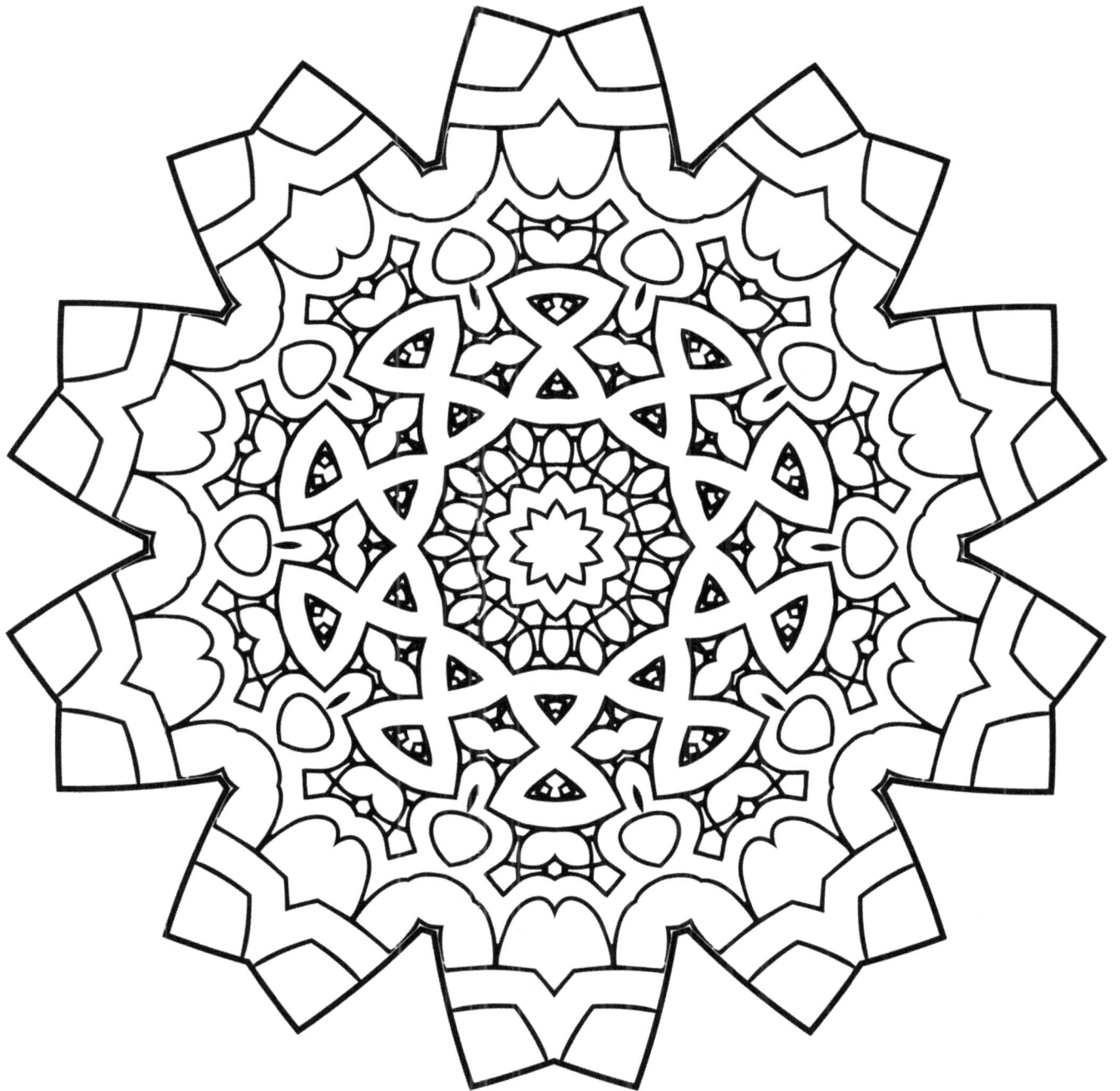

Date Completed: _____

Media Used:_____

_____

_____

Notes: _____

_____

_____

_____

_____

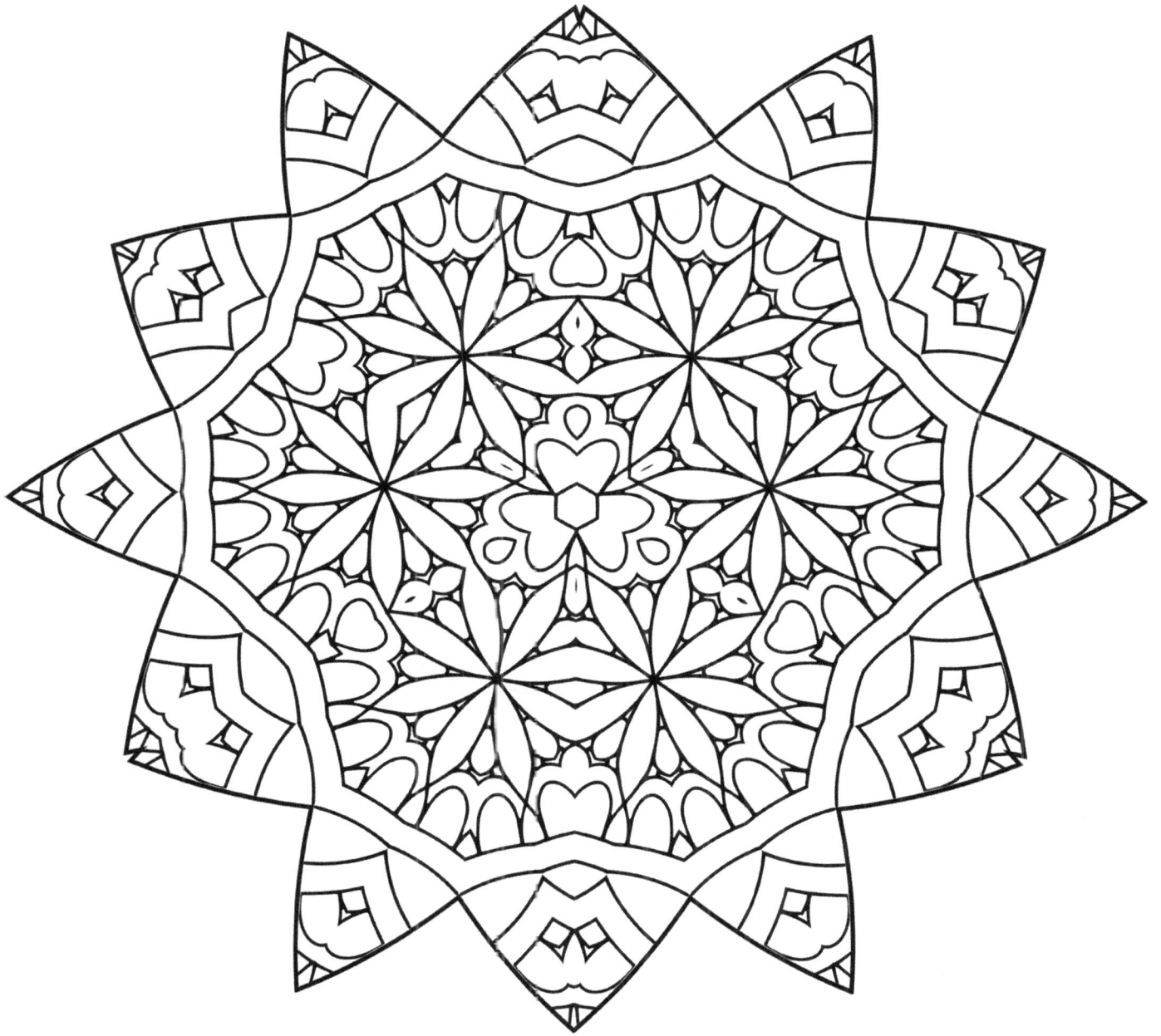

Date Completed: _____

Media Used:_____

_____

_____

Notes: _____

_____

_____

_____

_____

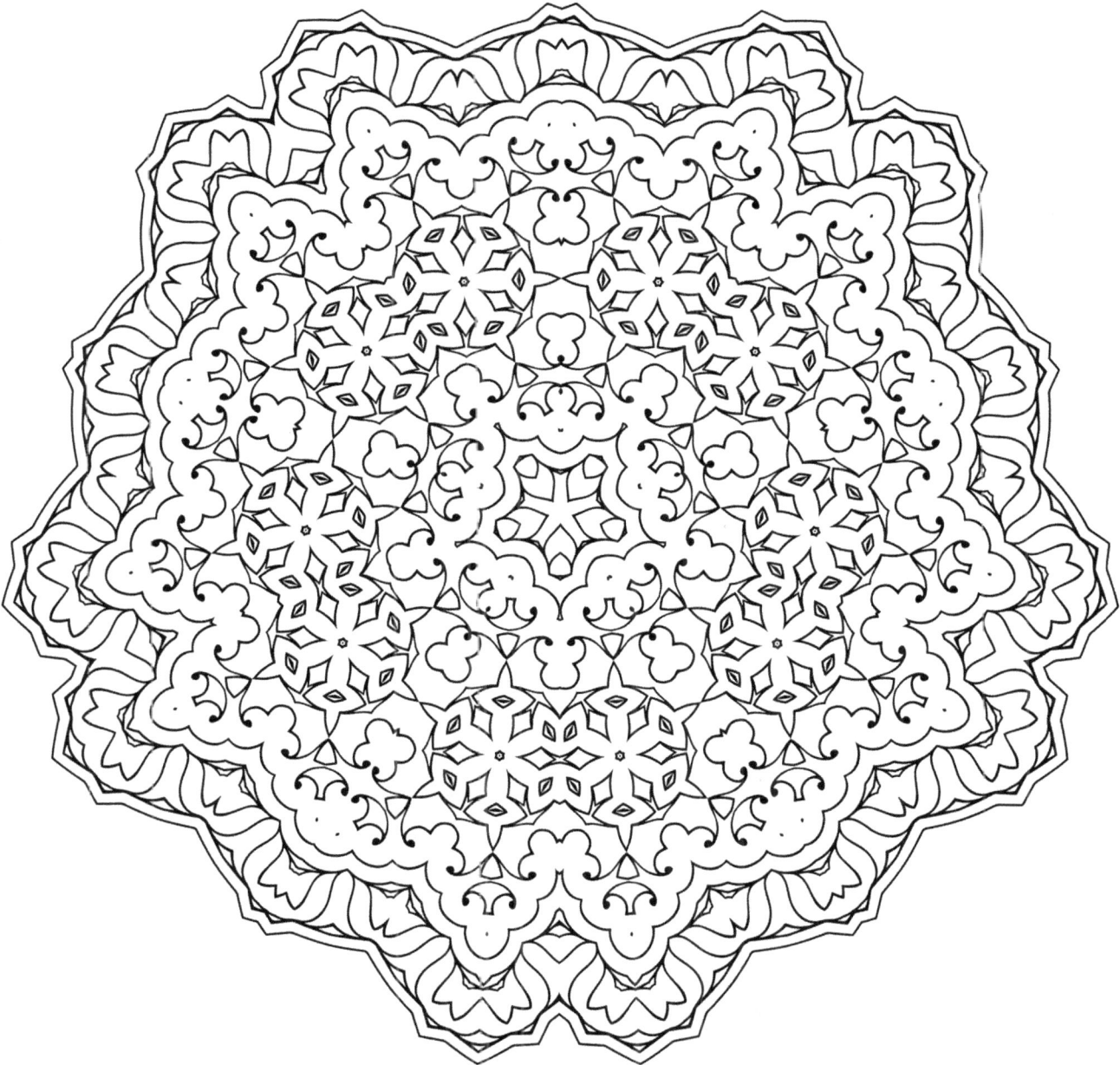

Date Completed: _____
Media Used:_____
_____
_____
Notes: _____
_____
_____
_____
_____

About the Author

Dr. Deb Gilbert has been working from home since 2007 and is an online professor of education, research, and leadership. She has been involved in public schools and higher education for over 25 years and has a passion for promoting literacy. She is the author of several books, journals, and adult coloring books.

For more information on Deb Gilbert, please join her at
www.hellerbrotherspublishing.com
and on Facebook at:
https://www.facebook.com/journalsforyou/

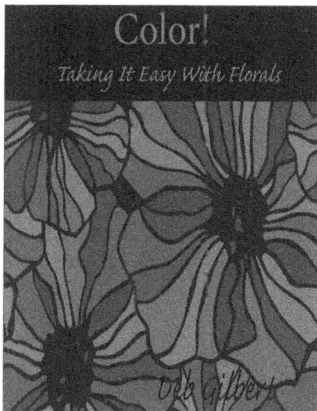

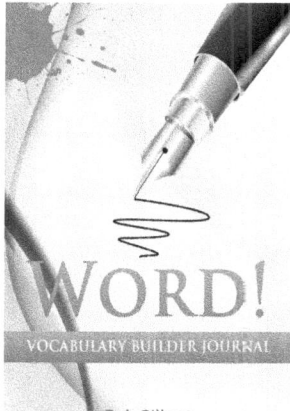

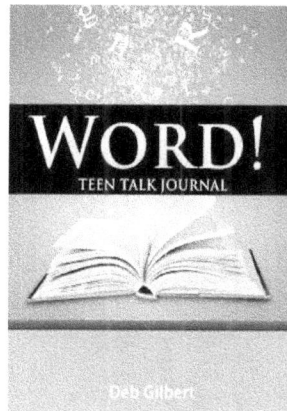

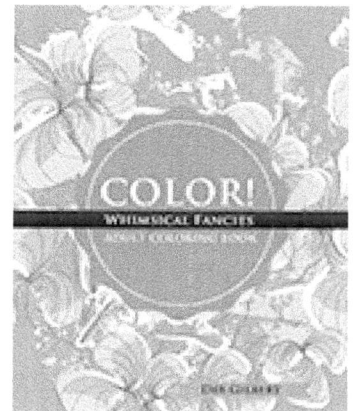

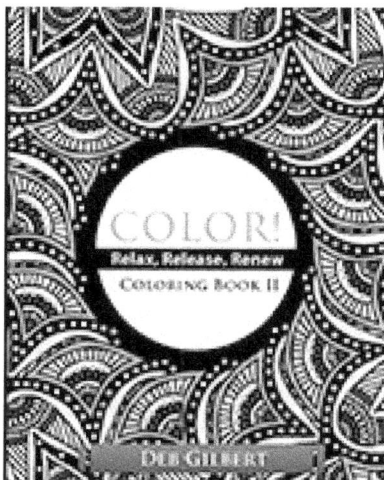

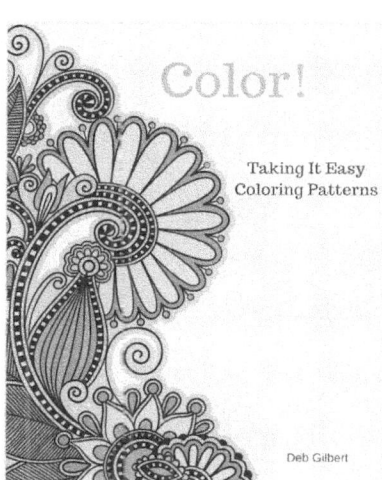

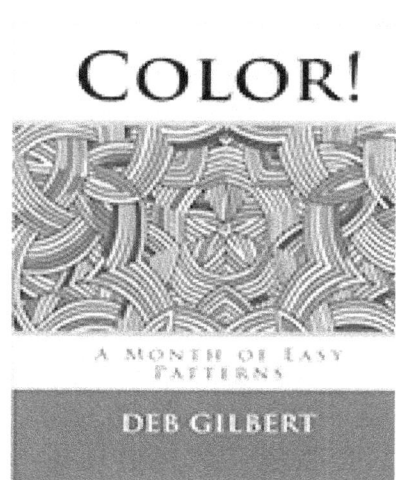